Also from Westphalia Press
westphaliapress.org

The Idea of the Digital University

Dialogue in the Roman-Greco World

The Politics of Impeachment

International or Local Ownership?: Security Sector Development in Post-Independent Kosovo

Policy Perspectives from Promising New Scholars in Complexity

The Role of Theory in Policy Analysis

ABC of Criminology

Non-Profit Organizations and Disaster

The Idea of Neoliberalism: The Emperor Has Threadbare Contemporary Clothes

Donald J. Trump's Presidency: International Perspectives

Ukraine vs. Russia: Revolution, Democracy and War: Selected Articles and Blogs, 2010-2016

Iran: Who Is Really In Charge?

Stamped: An Anti-Travel Novel

A Strategy for Implementing the Reconciliation Process

Issues in Maritime Cyber Security

A Different Dimension: Reflections on the History of Transpersonal Thought

Contracting, Logistics, Reverse Logistics: The Project, Program and Portfolio Approach

Unworkable Conservatism: Small Government, Freemarkets, and Impracticality

Springfield: The Novel

Lariats and Lassos

Ongoing Issues in Georgian Policy and Public Administration

Growing Inequality: Bridging Complex Systems, Population Health and Health Disparities

Designing, Adapting, Strategizing in Online Education

Secrets & Lies in the United Kingdom: Analysis of Political Corruption

Pacific Hurtgen: The American Army in Northern Luzon, 1945

Natural Gas as an Instrument of Russian State Power

New Frontiers in Criminology

Feeding the Global South

Beijing Express: How to Understand New China

Demand the Impossible: Essays in History as Activism

A New Art of Brewing Beer, Ale, and Other Sorts of Liquors

So as to Render Them More Healthfull to the Body and Agreeable to Nature, and to Keep Them Longer From Souring, With Less Trouble and Charge Then Generally Practised, Which Will Be a Means to Prevent Those Torturing Distempers of the Stone, Gravel, Gout, and Dropsie: Together With Easie Experiments for Making Excellent Drinks With Apples, Currans, Goodberries, Cherries, Herbs, Seeds, and Hay &c., and the Way to Preserve Eggs Five or Six Months From Being Musty or Rotten: Wih an Appendix How to Make Fruit Trees Constantly Fruitful: Also a Way How Every One May Purge Themselves With Common Salad Herbs and Roots, and a Method How to Prevent Constiveness in the Body

by Thomas Tryon

WESTPHALIA PRESS
An Imprint of Policy Studies Organization

A New Art of Brewing Beer, Ale, and Other Sorts of Liquors

Westphalia Press
An imprint of Policy Studies Organization
1527 New Hampshire Ave. NW
Washington, D.C. 20036
info@ipsonet.org

ISBN-13: 978-1-63391-837-5
ISBN-10: 1-63391-837-8

Cover design by Jeffrey Barnes:
jbarnesbook.design

Daniel Gutierrez-Sandoval, Executive Director
PSO and Westphalia Press

Updated material and comments on this edition
can be found at the Westphalia Press website:
www.westphaliapress.org

A NEW

A R T

OF

BREWING

Beer, Ale, and other ſorts of *Liquors,* ſo as to render them more healthful to the Body, and agreeable to Nature, and to keep them longer from ſouring, with leſs Trouble and Charge then generally practiſed, which will be a means to prevent thoſe torturing Diſtempers of the *Stone, Gravel, Gout* and *Dropſie.*

Together with eaſie Experiments for making excellentDrinks with *Appies, Currans, Gooſberries, Cberries, Herbs, ſeeds,* and *Hay,&c.* And the way to preſerve *Eggs* five or fix Months from being Muſty or Rorten. With an *Appindix* how to make Fruit-trccs conſtantly fruitful.

Alſo a way how every one may purge them themſclvcs with common Salad Herbs and Root. And a Method how to prevent Coſtiveneſs in the Body.

Recommended to all Brewers, Gentlemcn, and others that brew their own Drink.

Bythe Author of the *Way to Long Life, Health,* and *Happineſs,* &c.

Liceaſed,and *Entered according to Order.*

London, Prinrcd for *Tho. Salusbury* at the Sign of the *Temple at Temple-Bar in Fleet ſtreet, 1690.*

A NEW ART OF Brewing, ect.

THO I have *no* other Deſign, in reſpect of Brewers, then only, to ſave them a great deal of Pains, and no ſmall part of their daily Charge, and towardſ the reſt of Mankind, but an honeſt moſt charitable Intention of advertizing them what may conduce, both to tho Health of their Bodies,Tranquility of their mind and Advantage of their eſtates; yet I am not ſo Ignorant of the Worlds common uſage, as not to expect, that offering to Diſſwade from certain inveteral (but miſchievous) Cuſtoms, I am like to meet with no leſs than Hate or Reproach, or at leaſt Scorn and Contempt, from the greateſt part of thoſe, whoſe welfare I would gladly promote. However, as the Conſcience of my own Innocence, and certain Experience and Knowledge of the the Truth, of what I Recommend will be a ſuffcient Buckler againſt all the Darts of Envy, Ingraritude, Noife Noiſe and Folly :So I do not Deſſpair, but this ſmall Treatiſe may have the happineſs to meet with ſome few, to little wedded to Tradition and their own Humours, as to be willing to hearken to the Dictates ofWiſdom, Reaſon, and Nature, wherever they meet them, or through communicatied in an homely manner, by a very week and inperfecr Inſtrument, Methinks there ſhould ſearce be any man that hath ever entertained his Thoughtſ for one half hour, in a ſerious Conſiderarion of his own Structure, and how and by what Natural means he doth ſubſiſt in this World, but muſt have taken notice, that as the Subſtance of our Bodies ſufers a daily Expence, Decay, or Wafling, as well by the action of our own innate (or inbread hear) prefpiration of Spirits, and the more pure parts of the Humours. thorow the pores of the Skin, impreffions of the Ambient Air, as by the common and more grofs Evacuations ; fo there is reqired a daily fupply of Nourifhment to repair and make good what foever if thus fpent of the Store which provided to fupport and preferve the Microcofm.

To this End, as outwardly the All-wife and moft Bountiful Creator has prepared variety of excellent Foods and Liquors; fo inwardly he has both given us Reafon, Wifdom, and Knowledge (if we wilt hearken to and exert it) to diftinguifh which of them are at all times beft and moft requifite for us; as alfo fixed the Members and Organs of our Bodies, in their feveral places and offices, to be affifting and fubfervient to each other, in order to the effecting of this admirable Work.

Of thefe the Stomach is the firft and principal Agent, which as it were a Kitchin ferves to drefs and prepare all Meats that are brought into it, and by its Concocting Facylty redufes them into a white milky Subftance, which is called *Chyle,* which paffing thence throughout the lower Orifice of the Stomach into the Intrails, having there but a flow paffage (by reafon of many turnings and windings, by which the Guts are mutually inclofed and united to the Mefentery) *it* if further digefted and feperated, and the purer part by the Meforaick Veins (called the Hands of the Liver) is thorough the Veins (from the Office called *Vena Porta*) carried into the hollow parts of the Liver, whereby a higher and more elaborate Concoction is turned into that admirable Balfamick Liquor, called *Blood.*

This Blood paffes from thence into the *Vena Cava,or* great hollow Vein, whofe Trunk divides itfelf into two large Branches, the one tending downwards to carry blood to the lower parts; the other upwards, and mounteth even to the Throat, dividing again by the way into other Branches, one of which fafteneth it felf to the right Ventricle of the Heart, by which the blood iſ brought thither from the Liver, where being yet higher elaborated and inriched, 'tis tranſ muted or carried over to the left Ventricle,where the Arteries takes their original, which contains the Vital Blood and Spirits, whoſe Office it is to enliven and exerciſe the Faculties of the Body.

By other Branches it ariſeth into the Brain, where the Animal Spirits are made, being the Seat of Phanſie, Reaſon, Judgment, and Memory (which noble Faculties by thoſe Spirits are exerciſed) as alſo of all Senſe and Motion; for from the Brain areall the Nerves (or Sinews) divided into all the parts, which cauſe a voluntary Motion in the Body, by which it walks, ſtands, lyes down, labours, riſes, or uſeth any other Exerciſe, according to the Dictes of the Will, which cannot be done without the miniſtry of the Nerves.

Thus you ſee the whole economy of Narure, how, what is received at the Mouth is turned into Chyle by the Stomach, that Chyle into Blood by the Liver. Of the purer parts of the Blood are made Vital Spirits by the Heart, and Animal Spirits by the Brain, all which being thorow the Veins and Arteries (like ſo many Channels or Conduict Pipes) convcycd to the principal Member, and from thence by abundance of ſmaller Veſſels into every part of the Body, Growth and Vigour at leaſt, a continual and ſuitable Supply ought to be thereby communicated to the whole.

But if what is taken into the Body, that is, our Meats and Drinks, be either improper in quality, or too great in quantity, it does in either caſe diſturb this curious ecnomy, and fruſrate Natures Intentions and Operations ; for as unwholſom Meats and Drinks muſt needs give an unwholſome Nouriſh ment (the Effects always precipitating quality conſentaneous to its Cauſes) and every thing delighteth to produce its Smile's, ſo if the Errors be only in quantity (which tho' too frequent, yet rarely happens without the other) the Conſequence is ſtill worſe, Exceſs in Eating and Drinking laying the Foundations of almoſt all Diſeaſes; for ſcarce could the Starry Influences, Injuries of Inſalubrious Air, various Seaſons of the Year and the like External Accidents,have power to beget Diſeaſes, unleſs the Body were prediſpoſcd to receive their Effects by ill Humours, is the Reſult of Indigeſtions,and originally cauſed from the Faculties of the Stomach being abaſed and perverted ; for when the Stomach is nautiated with diſagreable Food or Drink, or over-charged with Exceſsſ, it cannot conceal and turn ſuch Matters into good Chyle(but not being able to contain it long) thorow ill Crude, as it iſ into the Intrails, which being alſo oppreſſed, cannot ſo ſpeedily conveigh thorow them the indigeſted load, but it receiveth there an impcrfet alteration, and ſo is by the Veins of the Meſentery drawn away to the Livcr, which being likewiſe indiſpoſed at the rcceipt of fuch unprepared Matter, is as unable to convert the unequal Maſs into good Blood, but thruſts it out into the larger Veins, mixed and infected with evil

Humours, and from thence to the Heart the Seat of Life, (which like a Lamp almoſt drown'd with Oyl) is even ſtifled and overcome ; thence alſo it is carried to the Brain (the Fountain of Senſe and Motion) which being clouded with Vapors and ſuperfluous Humours, its Faculties are interrupted, the briſk and active Phanſie clogged and dulled, Reaſon mudled, and Judgment vitiated, and all the admirable Storehouſe of Memory oppreſſed and confounded; from theſe nobler Parts and larger Veſſel, it iſ throghout the ſmall ones ſpread all over the Body, every part taking its unhappy ſhare, and by reaſon of the want of its due Concoction in the principal Members, cannot give due Nouriſhment to thoſe parts remote; but by theſe Errors often repeated, the Harmony of Nature is every where diſturbed, and the whole Body made a Magazin of corrupt Humours, which (like home-bred Traitors in a City) are continually ready to let in fierce and cruel Diſeaſes upon the leaſt External Attack, or (if that be wanting) will from their own Malignity (as Domeſtick Rebellions and Inſurrections are cauſed in ill govern'd States) creates Diſturbances within, endangering the peace both of Body and Mind,and even threatning Subverſion to the Throne of Life. By what has been ſaid, it appears of what vaſt Importance, due Conſidereti0n, and Caution in our Meats and Drinks is, not only for the Securing Health of Body, Prevention of Diſeaſes,bur alſo in order to the obtaining Serenity of Mind and Calm Affections, and the improving all our Intellectual Faculties, 'tis an old Rule, *The Paſſions of the Mind follow the Temperatement of the Body;* for ſuch Diet as you uſe, ſuch will be your Blood; and aſ your Blood iſ pure, or impure, ſuch will be your Spirits, Natural,Vital, and Animal , and conſequcntly all Functions and Operations of Body and Mind ſhall ſuitably be altered. Take a man never ſo modeſt, juſt and peaceble, let him over-charge himſelf with ſtrong Liquor, what a ſtrange Metamorphize, altogether incredible, did, not the lamentable freq-uency convince us, ſhall it make, as if ſome Body had ſtoln away the Man, and left a Beaſt,or rather a Devil in his ſhape; ſo do we not daily ſee, that thoſe who addict themſelves to Gluttony (tho' not ſo ſoon, yet in time as certainly as the other) loſe their Parts, and of ſharp, witty, judicious Perſons, become Fools and ſtupid Sots : But of the Inconveniences of improper Foods, and Exceſs even in the moſt Innocent, I have even at large Treated in other of my Writ-ings; not omitting, as occaſionally, to ſay ſomething thereof here: but the main Scope of thiſ preſent Treatiſe ſhall relate to Drink, and ſome particular Foods, that may be proper for ſuch as are afflicted with the Stone and Gravel, and alſo the Sorts they ought to forbear (not ſo much to ſhew the odiouſneſs of that Swiniſh ſin, Drunkenneſs, nor in admoniſhing thoſe who think themſelves, and are by others numbred amongſt the moſt ſober, that even they are guilty of great Exceſs in the quantity of

Liquor, as well as in the quality, which through ill Cuſtoms they ſwallow down beyond the neceſſity of Nature) but eſpecially to take notice of the ill quality of thoſe Liquorſs that are uſed by moſt People, ariſing from their undue Prepara- tions, and to ſhew both the Reaſons how and why the ſame do breed diſeaſes in Human Bodies; as alſo to offer Remedies whcreby the ſame may be prevented, and Drink truly refreſhing, exhilerated, and friendly to Nature, made and accommodated to General Uſe.

The firſt ſtep towards the Generation of the Stone and Gravel, and alſo the Gout, Conſumption, and various other Diſeaſes of the like Nature, is the Frequent drinking of ſtrong, hot, ſharp, intoxicating ſtale Liquors, and fiery prepared Drinks, as Beer high boyled with Hops, Brandy, Rum, old Wines, eſpecially Claret and Whitewine, which for the moſt part tend towards a Spirit, *(viz.)* Heat and Sharpneſs, becoming its predominating quality, all ſuch Drinks do, in ſuch Conſtitutions by Simile, contract and generate in the Paſſages and Ureters a hard gretty Subſtance, and of a mixt Saturnine Martial Nature , which is the firſt principle and beginning of the Diſeaſe called the *Stone,* and all its Symptoms and Attendances. Nor is that the only Evil thereby occaſioned in the Human Nature, for ſuch Liquors do too violently ſtir up and evaporate the pure eſ- ſential Spirits, and as it were burn up the ſweet Oyl or Humour *Radicallis,* the Balſom of Life, whereby the Blood becomes Infected with a ſharp hot quality, and its free Circulation is obſtructed, which Cauſes unnatural or burdenſom heat in all the External Parts, and lays the Seeds of various Diſtempers, according to the Nature of each. Conſtitution, Country; and Clymate, as Conſumtions, Palſies, Fevers, Gout, Stone, and the like.

Secondly, It is alſo to be noted and conſidered,the boyling of Hops two, three, or four hours in Beer, is a thing of a pernicious Conſequence, tho' it be unadviſed, and ignorantly practiſed, they falſly imagine that there Drink will be come the better thereby; whereas indeed they do by that Error, in a great. meaſure, evaporate or ſuffocate thc pure Spirits, which are the Preſervers of the ſweet frindly Baſamick Body, in all things whence the amiable, meek,or mild opening quality do exiſt, which whilſt any thing remain intire or unviolated, is the Moderater and Qualificr, or the harſh, bitter, aſtringent Nature ; therefore Hops and Beer ſo boyled do prove very injurious to ſeveral Conſtitutions; for after Drink is thus prepared, the predominant quality in it is, hot, fulſom, ſtrong, and bitter; and of a reſtringent Nature and Operation, prejudicial to Health eſpecially to all ſuch perſons, who by their Conſtitutions are ſubject or inclinablc unto the Stone or Gravel.

Thirdly, It is further to be conſidered, That the boyling of Wort, or any Spirituous Liquor that iſ drawn or extracted from things, whoſe Body iſ opened by Firmentation, as Mault is in a vegy high degree, does not only deſtroy and evaporate the fine, thin, ſubtle Spirits and Quality, which are only capable of Penetration, but it does, as it were, fix or ſtagnate the whole, by which it becomes of a groſſer, fuller, or ſtronger taſte in the Mouth,which through Uſe, Cuſtom, and Ignorance is eſteemed a Vertue or Strength ; but the contrary is to be underſtood ; for thereby it becomes of a heavier Operation, lies longer in the Stomach, ſending groſs Fumes and Vapours into the Crown, and Seldom fails to obſtruct the Paſſages, becauſe it hath loſt great part of thoſe fine penetrating properties, which is eaſily demonſtrated to your Senſes; *(viz.)* Unboyled Wart hath a fine pleaſant ſweetneſs in taſte, and it is of an opening, cleanſing quality and operation; and then taſte or drink ſome of the ſame Wort boyled with or without Hops, and you will find that this laſt hath not only loſt its pleaſant taſte and ſweetneſs, but alſo its opening penetrating Virtues, by which it becomes of another Nature and Operation; which Fermentation does in ſome degree help, but it cannot regain thoſe fine, thin, penetrating Virtues and Spirits, that it hath loſt in the boyling, the fierce heat of the fire, being an utter Enemy to all ſpirituous Drinks, Liquors, or Cordials. It is alſo to be noted, that unboyled Beer or Ale do generally drink ſmaller in the Mouth then that which is boyled, becauſe its ſpirituous, ſweet qualities are not ſo much deſtroyed, ſuffocated, or ſtagnated by the fiery heat of the fire, as the other, but it moſt naturally warms the Stomach, and not ſo ſubject to ſend Fumes into the Head, and runs quicker thorow the Body, purges more powerfully by Urine, which are naturally Teſtimonies of its Virtues, and that the better Parts are preſerved in the preparation. AIſo it is further to be conſidered That all ſorts of Dunks made without fire, alt ho' with raw crude Fruits, Apples, Grapes, and the like, as Wine, Syder, and many other ſorts, are not only more ſpirituous and briſker in operati on, but alſo more cleanſing and penetrating, if order and temperance be obſerved. But note that all ſorts of fermented Drinks are much better and greater prcſer vers of Health when new,then old or ſtale, for Age does naturally conſume and turn the mild, ſoft, ſweet, opening, healing Virtues, into a hard , keen property; for this cauſe all ſtale Beer, old Wine, and Sider, are far hotter in operation than new, and conſequently more prejudicial to Health, eſpecially to all ſuch as are naturally ſubject to the Stone, Gravel, Gout, or Conſumption, for it over-hears the Blood, and conſumes the Radical Moiſture; not but that the new Wine, Syder, Beer or Ale,are endued with as great a quantity of Spirits as the old, as is manifeſt in Diſlillation: But ſo long aſ the mild, ſweer, opening Virtues remain intire, ſtrong, and powerful, this harſh fire, keen or ſharp Spitit, is thereby moderated, qualified, or allayed by the ſweet Imbraces of thoſe friendly Virtues; which friendly quality, Age turns into heat, ſharpneſs, and kenenels, as is moſt clearly manifeſted in firmenting of all ſweet Bodies, which no Art can cure or bring back, it being eaſie by the help of the fiery Art to deſtroy all the mild, opening , friendly Properties of each thing, and turn or tranſmute them into their Original, *viz.* into a hot, ſtrong Spirit, but when this is done, there is no further *Progreſs* to be made, for it then ſtands in its original Qualities, and will admit of no cure ; thereforc it is eaſie to deſtroy, but hard to make alive, eſpecially in all Fire Operations ; and remember this, that whenſoever any violence is offered to any thing, more eſpecially to things that has paſſed thorough firmentation, that the beſt and friendly Virtues do firſt ſuffer Injury, or Prejudice, which every one ought to underſtand, firſt in themſelves, and ſecondly in all other things, more eſpecially in all Pre parations by Fire; therefore ſuch as would drink Beer or Ale more wholſom, may, unleſs they be too old to learn, and too obſtinate to be taught, obſerve the Rules following, which will make your Drink wholſomer, and ſave you both trouble and charge ; and if neither Profit nor Regard to Health can wean you from the ſlavery of ſilly old Cuſtom, your Underſtandings are certainly miſerable already, and no wonder if your Bodies prove ſo in a little time.

Firſt, Make your Water or Liquor neer boyling hot, then put juſt ſo much into your Maſhtub as will wet your Mault, ſtir it, and let it ſtand half an hour, which will diſpoſe the Mault the better to give forth its Virtues and Sweetneſs into the Liquor; then add your whole quantity of Water or Liquor to your Mault that you purpoſe to put up the firſt time, then let it ſtand one hour and a half; but if you would have your firſt Wort very ſtrong then two hours, if the Seaſon be not hot; then put what a quantity of Hops you think convenient into your Receiver, and let your Wort run to them, and after your Hops have infuſed an hour and half in your Wort, then ſtrain it off in your Coolers; you have done with your firſt Wort. Then put upon your Mault your ſecond Liquor near the ſame Heat as the firſt, rather cooler if any difference; but this muſt ſtand on your

Mault but one hour at moſt; then take what quantity you pleaſe of freſh Hops and put into your Receiver as before, and let your ſecond Wort run to them; then take both ſecond Wort and Hops together and put into your Coppcr, there let them infuſe till your Wart is near boyling, but not boyl; then ſtran this alſo into you Coolers, which you have done with alſo. Now ifyou would inlarge your quantity, which is not proper, which in its due place I ſhall demonſtrate, then put up what quantity you think convenient of cold Water, and let it ſtand, not more then half an hour, and then run it off to ſome freſh Hops, and then put this third Wort, and alſo Hops, into thc Copper, as you did the ſecond, and let the Hops infuſe till they are near boy ling, then ſtrain it off into your Coolers, and you have done; but you muſt remember that your Liquor or Watcr do not boyl, for boy ling of Water does irritate and evaporate the ſubtle fine panetrating Spirits, whence the more friendly, mild, opening qualities do exiſt, which do make ſuch Water or Liquor more harſh, hard and fixed, which do render it not ſo capable to draw forth or extract the ſweet virtues of the Mault; for boyling of Water does open its Body, and ſets the Spirit on the wing ; for this cauſe all Water that hath been boyled becomes of a colder, harſher , and harder nature then that which never bcen fired and thereore it will not prepare any Foods and Drinks ſo natural, not to that advantage as that which hath not been boyled. And that you may be convinced of this Truth, boyl a quantity of good River water, and put it into a good clear Veſſel, and let it ſtand awhile , and thcn take a like quantity and put into another Veſſel , and let that ſtand the ſame time as the other, and you will find the boyled Water to ſtink, and never be ſweet again; but your Water which remains intire, not touched with thc fire, will alſo ſtink, or rather firment , but then it will be ſwcet andgood as for any uſe as before; the Rcaſon thereof is this, for the Fire doth force forth and evaporate the eſſential Spirits and good preſerving Virtues, which do render of a dead, dull, phlegmatick, groſs Nature and Operation, as we have more largely Diſcourſed in our *Way to Health*.

Secondly It is a general Cuſtom to put up hot Liquor a third time on your Mault, or rather Grains, and to let it ſtand an hour or more, which makes a very ill ſort of Drink; for the firſt and ſecond Liquors have extracted ordrawn forth all the briſk, lively, ſweet qualities of the Mault, ſo that this third hot Liquor hath nothing to work on, or draw forth, but only a groſs Subſtance, ſtinking, harſh, bitter, or keen quality, void of all the ſeminal or ſweer Virtues.Now if there be any goodneſs left in the Mault or Grains, it is weakandfainty, and the groſs, fulſom, Martial, Saturnine Properties are ſtrong. and have obtained the Aſcendant, and therefore they do in a moment ſwallow up the fading Virtue, and tranſmute it into its own Property; for theſe fiery qualities do, with open Jaws, devour the friendly virtues, and turn them into their own Nature, *(viz.)* into a fiery keen quality, a meer *Caput mortum* Phlegm ; for all things when they have attained their higireſt degree, limit, or perfection,do by degrees, as it were, go backwards, and ſink towards their Original or Root whence theӱ proceeded.

Thirdly, By what hath been ſaid it appears, and ought to be conſidered, That the ſame Beer that iſ made of the third putting up of the Liquor on the Mault or Grains, is generally pernicious to Health : foras is mentioned before, the firſt and ſecond Liquors, have before drawn forth all or moſt of the good, ſweer, friendly Virtues, and there remains nothing but a dull, heavy, groſs Phlegm of a tart, ſour Nature, which in- corporates with the Liquor, and is of a very unpleaſing taſte ; and ſmall, and then the common Cuſtom is to take this third Wort, (indeed not fit for Hoggs-waſh) and boyl it ſtoutly with the Dregs of the Hops which hath been boyled ſeveral hours before in the firſt and ſecond Wort, which ſtill doth more increaſe the Miſchief; for the boyling of Hops totallt ſuffercates, evaporates, and deſtroys all the volatile Spirits and ſoft friendly Virtues, and there does nothing remain in them after ſuch boyling, but an harſh, bitter, aſtringent ſour Property, which ſuch ſmall Wort in the boyling draws forth.

For this cauſe moſt ſmall Beer, eſpecially that which iſ made after Ale or ſtrong Beer, is injurious to Health, and the common drinking thereof does generate various Diſeaſes, but more eſpecially the Scurvy in the Blood ; therefore all that do regard their Health,ought to forbear drinking ſuch ill prepared Liquors. The beſt Small, or Table Beer, is to be made by adding a large proportion of Liquor to your Mault (according as you would have it) and then mix the firſt and ſecond Wort equally together,for the Reaſons before mentioned, for all Preparations were intended to open the crude Body by firmentation, or ſome other way, which do not only awaken, and ſet the fine Spirits and friendly Virtues on the wing, but alſo in ſome degree excite the harſh, bitter, ſour, aſtringent Properties, but ſtill the balſamick Virtues are moſt volatile, and readieſt to give forth themſelves, when communicated to a proper *Minſtrim,* as appears not only in the Art of Brewing, but alſo in common Chymiſtry the Spirits and good Properties gives forth the them-ſelves,and runs off firſt, and afterwards the bitter, aſtringent, ſour, harſh ones follows.

Fourthly,The quantity of Hops for Beer, if you propoſe to keep it half a year, or a year, ought to be ſix or ſeven pound to eight Buſhels of Mault, and ſo proportionable ; but for Beer or Ale that is to be ſpent preſently, two, three, or four to eight Buſhels will ſuffice. Alſo note, That all ſorts of Beer or Ale are beſt new, and much more agreeable to Nature, as I have mentioned before ; for the longer any firmented Drinks are kept , the more they tend towards harſhneſſs, keneneſs, and ſharpneſs, and the Saturnine, Martial Propertieſ are thereby advanced, and the mild, friendly qualities debilitatedt, for which reaſon all ſtale Beer does heat the Body, and much more diſorder it then new.

Fifthly, Another thing is in a moſt ſpecial manner to be noted, *(viz)* That your Veſſels in which you cool your Wort, ought to be well cleanſed ; and alſo your Maſhtub (*viz.*) waſhed well with cold water, which iſ better than hot; for boyling water does, as it were, fright or drive back into the wood a certain , ſour, fulſom quality that the former Wort left behind and which the wood of the Coolers had ſuckt in; for the humidity or ſwcet quality that the wood receives from the Wort, do preſently turn very ſharp, ſour, and keen, eſpecially in hot Seaſons of the Year, ſo that when the freſh, new, ſweet Wort comes into ſuch Coolers, it does moſt eagerly and powerfully attract and draw forth that lurking keen, ſharp, ſour quality, that the wood had received and retained, which will occaſion the whole to become of a ſharp quality, which is called *(Pricks,)* but hardly perceivable to the Palate; but when it iſ firmented,this evil quality gets the Aſcendent over the whole, which is the principal occaſion why Brewers Ale in hot Seaſons will not keep above four, five, or ſix days, or there abouts. Now the beſt way to prevent this Evil is,that your Coolers are ſtill waſhed well in cold water, wherein ſome bitter Herbs or Seeds are infuſed 24 hours, as *Wormwood* gathered and dried, as we have taught in our *Way to Health;* and after they are well cleanſed with this bitter watcr,then expoſe your Veſſels to the open Air as much as poſſible you can, for nothing ſweetens and cleanſeth ſo much as Air; alſo avoid putting your Veſſels into Cellars,or any cloſe Places where theAir hath not its free influences. The like is to be done in th cleanſing your Tun in which you work your Drink in. The like is to be underſtood in Ovens; for if you bake ſpicy Foods, as Pies, and the like, and afterwards heat the Oven for ſmall Bread, ſuch Bread will be tinged, and ſmell ſtrong of the former things, that is, if the Oven be heat preſently; but if the Oven ſtands open two or three days, in which time thoſe ſpicy qualities will evaporate; for the Spirits of things are ſo quick, powerful, and ſubtile, that thcy penetrate even the hardeſt of Bodies,which neither fire nor water can preſently extinguiſh, but they remain as it were intire and fixed,until a ſutable ſubject matter be offered, into which, as by Simile, they retreat, and therewith readily incorporate, and therefore remember your Friend the Air; and to prevent this and many other Inconveniences, expoſe your Veſſels to its freeInfluences; for no Element hath ſo great power to cleanſe, ſweeten, and to give true Lifc to every thing, according to the nature of each, as *Air;* arid where it has its free Circulation and Influence, it deſtroys all Putrifation, Vermine,and evil Scents. But becauſe brewing is become a Trade, and ſuch muſt brew three or four days in a week, therefore they have not ſufficient time to expoſe their Veſſels to this cleanſing Element, as Houſwives, and others, that brew only for their own private Families, it will therefore be convenient for them to Copper, Lead, or Tin their Coolers over, as alſo the Maſh-tub or Tin they firment or work there drink in, but Copper and Tin is beſt, which will in a great degree prevent the ſouring or pricking of their Ale in Summer, and their Beer will have the ſame advantage, for the ſweet Spirits cannot ſo eaſily penetrate thoſe hard Metaline Bodies, nor will ſo great a quantity of Humidity enter, and that which does will not become ſharp, nor ſour, as in wood, having no ſuch ſubject matter to work on.

It is alſo to be noted, That your Wort ought to ſtand very thin or ſhallow in your Coolers, for that will preſerve it from fretting and growing ſharp or keen, if the other Circumſtances before mentioned be obferved. Moreover,your Wort ought to be, as it were, quite cold, before it be put together to work, for if it be ſet together too hot, it will firment ſo violently, and in a moments time irritate and awaken the hot, ſharp, fiery Spirit, which ſhould not be ſtirred up, which ſpends and deſtroys the pure fine Spirit and ſweet Body, and conſequently cauſe your Beer or Ale to grow ſtale to faſt. Nor ought you when your Beer or Ale is in the Tun, to beat your Yeſt or Balm into it, as the Cuſtom of ſome Brewers is, eſpecially in and about *London,* which iſ very prejudicial to Health, and ought to be reſtrained by ſome Law; for this beating of the Yell into the drink does ſo mix, and as it were incorporate them together, and flatten or ſuffocate the fine penetrating Virtues, that in its firmentation the groſs excrementitious Matter cannot ſeperate from the finer Parts, by which means it does retain a ſtrong, groſs, and fulſom ſweetneſſ, which too many ignorant People admire, and count good and nouriſhing; but in truth ſuch Liquors fail not to ſur, foul,and obſtruct the Stomach and Paſſages, ſending dark dulling Fumes and vapors into the Head, and alſo generate an hard, gritty quality in People ſubject to the Stone and Gravel : Alſo ſuch Drinks are of evil conſequence to Women who are of tender Natures, and weaker Spitits and Heats than Men,therefore let them refrain the ſame, if they have any reſpect to their own and their Childrens Healths.

The ufual Courfe in brewing, is to let your Drink work in the Tun till it begins to fall or firment more gently, and then to Tun it up into your Casks, which new motion and agitation puts thc Drink upon a frefh firmentation, and caufes it oftentimes to work again as fierce and eagerly as it did at firft, or more,which is apt to make it fret or fpend it felf, for much or fierce working makes all Drinks to grow keen and ftale, fooner then when its firmentation is moderate. It will indeed in fuch Cafe become fine fomewhat fooner, becaufe the volatile Spirits and fweet Body is wafed, or rather turned into fharpnefs by, the two long and fierce firmenration. Therefore, thofe that have a mind to avoid this Inconveniency, ought to Tun or put up their Drink young, as the Brewerf calls it, that is, before it hath firmented too much, *(viz.)* fo foon as your Drink works you ought to Tun it into the Barrels or Vcffels, and you need not doubt but it will work fufliciently; nay, you may when your Wort is thorough cold, mix your Yeſt well with your Wort, and put it into your Veſſels preſently, and it will do extraordinary well.

Now if any think that ſo ſhort a time of Infuſion as I have preſcribed will not get out the Virtue and Goodneſs of the Hops without boyling of them ſtoutly, I anſwer, That all the mild, friendly virtues of Hops lycs as it were outward and ready, which with the leaſt violence are drawn forth, as appears by that delicate Scent and Odor which they caſt abaoad ; nay, ſo free and tender they are, that if they be not cloſe ram'd or ſtuffed into Baggs, the very Air Thall ſhall ſteal away moſt of their Excellency, and if ſo, what will the fierce heat and violent boyling do,which every conſiderate wiſe man ought to conſider;

Now as to the Nature of Hops, there is in them a moſt excellent glance or friendly opening quality, more eſpecially if they were dried in the Sun, which is to be preferred before the Hoſt or Kill; for the ſpirituous parts of this Plant is ſo nice,that it cannot indure any violent heat without prejudice to its fine Virtues,and you might almoſt as rationally make your Hay that way, which if you ſhould be ſo dull as not to perceive your folly, I doubt not but your bruit Beaſts would upbraid you of indiſcretion, and teach.you the diffrence. Hops naturally purges powerfully by Urine, if prepared and uſed with underſtanding, ſo that they are unjuſtly charged to breed the Stone; for, on the contrary, they are a ſpecial Remedy againſt it, if orderdered with judgment, and as they ought to be ; but as cvery thing conſiſts of Contraries, they may and do occaſion the Stone, and other Diſeaſes by accident ; but it is only when they are abuſed, and after their good Virtues are drawn off or evaporated by the force of fire,as boyling, and the like, which is done in a trice ; for no Herbs that have been dried as they ought, will endure the fire or boyling without manifeſt prejudice to the beſt Virtues; but it is a gentle Infuſion that will naturally,and without violence to Nature extract or draw forth all that is desired in Hops or any other dried or prepared Herbs; but 'tis true, it will not rouze nor infect your Liquor with their original harsh, bitter, fulsom, keen, hot Properties, which too many, for want of distinguishing the Principles of Nature, call Virtue and Strength; indeed Strength and Ficreenefs it is, but far from Virtue in respect of Human Bodies, nothing scarce being more inimical nnd injurious thereunto, which evil Properties in every thing are the more drawn Forth and increased by over much boyling, especially in Herbs and Vegitations which have been already firmented and digested by the Influencef of the Sun and Elements, whereby the gross phlemy Parts are opened, and the Spirits set upon the wing ready to come forth upon any gentle Summons.

But the swinging Objection is yet behind; You undertake (cries the professed Brewers, and the good 'Dames) to teach us to brew, yet leave out the principal Verb; you say the

Liquor, beforc it be put to the Mault, muſt only be moderately hot, not boyled: Well, ſuppoſe we ſhould yield to this, ſtill you forget to tell us, how long it ought to be boylcd after tis drawn off the Mault: Sure you would not have us brew without boyling at all, and make raw Ale and Beer, and take 12 or 16 s *per* Barrel only for a little Water bewitcht, the Rincings of a parcel of Mault and a few Hops in a little warm Water, with a ſmall doze of Yeſt to make it bubble in the Barrel, is like to make excellent humming Liquor. You complain of our Ale not keeping above a week; Is it poſſible (if unboy led) it ſhould keep at all? Nay, can Abſurdity call it Beer or Ale? He is like to have Cuſtomers, who ſhould write over his Sign, *Here's Beer and Ale to be ſold that never was boyled.* When the great fault that all the World finds with the Common Brewers Drink, is, that they do not boyl it half enough; and yet theyboyl it double the time as moſt Houſe-wives do. But if you could make good your words, *That good Ale and Beer might be made without boyling away a great quantiſſly of what they put up*, the Company of Brewers might well afford you Five hundred pounds a year for the Invention; for they could ſave almoft as much as their Exciſe comes to.

Anſwer. This I confeſs is the common Leiry, but it affects me no more than the buzzing of Flies about my Noſe in Autumn. The Objection conſiſts of ſeveral Parts, I will endeavour to anſwer them in order.

Firſt, As to the boyling of Wart after drawn from the Mault, I do aver that it is not only unneceſſary, but miſhievous, for the Reaſons before mentioned, and alſo by what follows Tis not boyling, but a due firm-entation that makes excellent generous Liquor. Wine and Sider are not boyled (at Leaſt not commonly) yet few People ſcruples, or think them ever the worſe: What's the Reaſon? becauſe they will ſay, the Grapes and Apples have paſſed through as much digeſtion aſ they ought, or need to have, by the ripening Influences of the Sun and Elements. Well then and what's the matter but ripe Barly which has not only received a far higher digeſtion by the ſame Sun and Elements, and will thereby remain good and ſound ſeveral years, which the beſt Grapes and Apples will not continue good a tenth part of the time; and though it be harder and more tenatious in its kind, has yet undergone a ſecond by its being made into Mault, and a third afterwards by our way of Infuſion in water, fitted to a due warmth to extract its ſpirituous Virtues and ſweet Body, ſhould need a fourth of boyling ſo long *as* you talk of. Is Water (ſeeing it is originally deſigned by God, and his Hand-maid Nature, the common Drink for all Creatures) of ſuch an illnature or quality, that it requires ſo much boyling? No certainly; for boyl a Gallon of Water to three quartſ, and let the remainder ſtand eight or ten days, and you'l find all its briſk pleaſantesſſ (before to any accuſtomed or undepraved pallat aſ reliſhing as any Liquor whatſoever) wholly loſt, ſo that you, or any

Beaſt, will nautiate to drink it. The Reaſons why we heat Water in brewing to ſuch a competent degree, is not ſo much to correct its Rawneſs, as they falſly call it, as to qualifie it to open and draw forth and imbibe the good virtues of the Mault, and ſo likewiſe of the Hops,which being once effected, all our pains in boyling is ſuperfluous, and not only ſo, but detrimental too; for henceforwards, if you proceed in your boyling, you do but raiſe and induce thoſe fierce bitter SpirIts in each thing or ingredient, which tho' fitly planted in them by Nature, for their own particular Conſervation, were yet never intended for the uſe of Man, as being injurious to his own Nature when unduly ſeperated from the friendly qualities or light of Nature. If then neither the Water, nor the Mault, nor the Hops require this tedious boyling, why iſ it practiſed? Or rather iſ it not a demonſtration, that the ſame is detrimental; ſince in all Nature's ways unneccifaries are hurtful, and over doing there (as well as in Morals) is a badge of Vice. You talk of Rawnefs, tis but raw that is indigefted (Argument) but the Drink I recommend is not fuch, fince it has paffed through all the digeftions and firmentations that it ought to do; and if People will not be willing to give 12. or 16 *s.* *per* Barrel for wholfom Drink, as for unwholfom, I can neither help nor hinder it, any more than perfwade an ignorant Irifh-man to quit his ftinking Butter (of as many Colours as the Rainbow) for wholfom, fweet Englifh Butter, which he counts hath no tafte in it; all this is but the effects of Cuftom. But add further, That this unboyled Drink will not keep; I anfwer (better for all good Intents) then your parboiled Geare. The beft way to prove a thing feafible is to do it: Now I have more than once made excellent Beer that never boiled, and yet has kept good, in your fenfe, a Twelve-month, and he that keeps any longer, has kept it fix Months too long. As for what is intended for long Sea Voyages, tis a particular bufinefs, and fo the boyling of it with Hops a great while may, together with excelſive ſalt meats, notably help the Seamen to the Scurvey, and yet both the one and the other might eaſily be avoided. But ſtill you urge, the only Fault all the world finds with Brewers of common Ale and Beer, that 'tis not boyled half enough,yet,and with as much Judgment, as once an honeſt Tubman, whoſe Imployment was to carry Beer and Ale from Brew-houres to his Maſters, whom I imployed to carry my Ale, who would needs be taſting: *Ay marry Maſter,* quoth he, *this is good Ale indeed, a man my taſte this is well boyled; if Brewers would but boil theirs ſo, we ſhould not have ſuch filthy unwholſom Drink in every Ale- houſe;* whilſt all the while the Ale he drank never boyled one wallop. But if I could make my words good, the Brewers might give me Five hundred pounds *per Annum,* and get mony by the bargain. I have made good my words, but I dare not undertake to rectifie at once all the debauched Palats and depraved Judgments throughout the Kingdom. If abundance of

People will love fulſom Ale, with Yeſt thwackt into it, to make it as they think ſtrong and mighty or the rueful Juices of parboyl'd Hops, and will Court the Stone, the Scurvey, the Conſumption and the like, to make work for the Sexton and thc Flanel Weavers, I can no more help it then the Self-murther of above 40000 a year, by the uſe of that Alamode Liquor, *Brandy*. And as for a Penſion from the Brewers, I am as far from ſeeking it, or (bleſs God) from needing it, as (I fear) they will be from following my well intended advice ; for it is no new thing for men,over whom Cuſtom and Tradition hathgot the Aſcendant, to not only againſt Reaſon, but even contrary to their own true Intereſt to. Much more I could ſay,but I think this enough for ſuch a Vulgar Objection.

Here give me leave to tell you, that there are a great number of brave Herbs and Vegitations that will do the buſineſs in brewing, as well aſ Hops, and for many Con-ſtitutions much better; for 'tis Cuſtom more than their real Virtues that renders Hops of general Uſe and Eſteem ; they are an excellent Herb, and would be much better if they were or could be dried in the Sun. Some other Herbs I ſhall here mention, fit to be made uſe of in Drinks.

Peny Royal and *Balm* are noble Herbs,and of excellent uſe in Beer or Ale; they naturally raiſe and cheer the drooping Spirits, and open and cleanſe the Paſſages after a friendly way, and with a mild Operations. And alſo they add great ſtrength and fragrancy, and makes brave, well taſted Drink, good toprevent and cure all, or moſt of thoſe Diſeaſes which the wiſe Ancients have appopriated that Herb unto. The like is to be underſtood of *Mint, Tanſte, Wormwood, Broom, Cardias, Century, Eye-Bright, Betony, Sage, Dadelion,* and good *Hay;* alſo many others, according to their Natures and Qfflalities, and for thoſe Diſeaſes to which they are reſpectively appropriated. But note, that all and every of theſe Herbs ought to be gathered in their proper Seaſons,and dry and preferved as we have given Directions in our *Way to Health;* for you ought nor to ufe any Herb or Vegitarion in Beer or Ale while they are green, except there be a neceffity.

Secondly, When you infufe in your Beer or Ale *Wormwood, Broom, Tanfey, Cardis,* or any other Herb that exceeds in birternefs, you ought nor to let them lye in your Wort above half an hour,or if you put in a good uanity, a quarter of an hour will be enough; for in all fuch bitter Hcrbs the Martial and Saturnine harfh Properties are near at hand, and the warw Wort will quickly ftir up and awaken their harfh, bitter, ftrong, aftringent qualities, which will prefently devour, fuffocate, and deftroy the fine fpirituous Virtues and opening clenfing Properties; and then fuch Drinks becomes of an hard, harfh,conftringent Nature, and are apt to obfruct the Stomach, and fend Fumes into the Head, heating the body and blood too violently ; therefore all, or moft Infufions of Herbs, made after this common way, more efpecially of bitter Herbs, are naughty and injurious to Health. As for Example ; They put a quantity of *Wormwood*, or ſome other bitter Herb, into their Beer or Ale, at or after it hath done working, and there let it lye infuſing (or rather rotting) two, three, four, five, or ſix Weeks, and in Ale-houſes ſo many Months, until the Caſk be out, whereby all the good; opening, penetrating, briſk Spirits, and fine Virtues of ſuch Herbs are totally deſtroycd, and inſtead thereof the Drink impregnated with their contraries, *(viz.)* with the harſh, bitter, churliſh, inimical Properties, eſpecially when ſuch Infuſions are made of *Wormwood;* for this reaſon common *Wormwood* Beer and Ale does not only hurt, but by degrees weaken the natural heat ot the Stomach, but ſends dulling Fumes and Vapors into the Head, and does prejudice the Eyes. Tis certain, Infuſion of Herbs, if due order be obſervcd, is the beſt and moſt profitableſt way yet found out to cbtain their Virtucs, both for common Uſe and Phyſick, far beyond Waters and Spirits drawn from them by Diſtillation, for thereby a burnIng, fierce, brimſtony Spirit is extracted, void of all the mild, cleanſing, opening Qualities or mild Virtues, which in firmentation are turned into a Degree of Anaſidity, which fits it, and renders it capable of Separation. As for Example, Take Sugar (which is the moſt balſamick and higheſt ſweet of any thing in the World) firmentation will in a little time turn the whole ſweet Body into a ſour, or a degree of ſharpneſs, then diſtil it, and you ſhall have a hot, burning Spirit,and for every pound of Sugar you will have near a pound of Spirit. Here you ſee the whole, ſweet, pleaſant Body is turned into a fierce, ſtong, burning Spirit, which has its uſes in Phyſick, but otherwiſe pernicious if commonly drunk, as too many do. The very ſame is to be underſtood in the firmenting and diſilling of any ſorts of Herbs; as in the Spirit of Scurvy-Graſs, ſo much of late cried up for its wonderful Virtues againſt the Scurvy, when in truth there is nothing in it ; for if you take Scurvy-Graſs, and infuſe it in

Brandy, or any other *Minſtrum,* for a certain time, till it firments to ſuch a degree, and then draw it off, or diſtil it; and inſtead then of obtaining the friendly, mild, cleanſing Virtues, and middle qualities, you have a ſtrong, fiery, brimſtony Spirit, which is not ſo good as rectified Spirit of Wine, and it hath no manner of force to cure or prevent the Scurvy in the Blood, for in good earneſt, the frequent uſe of ſuch Spirits do heat the Blood, obſtruct the Stomach, and increaſe Scorbutick Diſeaſes. The greateſt Virtues it hath, it being put into Ale, Beer, or Wine, in a Morning faſting, it quickens the Stomach, as Spirits do, and ſeems to purge by Urine, as moſt mixed Drinks do, eſpecially when Spirits are mixed with other Liquors, but it is the order and Time,and the Liquor it is put into, that is the principal point why it purges by Urine, being generally drunk in a Morning faſt ing, when the Stomach is free from Food, and the Paſſages leaſt obſtructed, then a Glaſs or two of any ſort of Liqqor or Drink will quickly run thorough a man, and purge much more by Urine, then at any other time ofthe day. And I do affirm, That if anyone take Brandy, or other good Spirits,and in a Morning fafting, drop fixty or feventy drops into a Glafs of Ale, and faft two or three houls after it, and it fhall purge by Urine, and alfo quicken the Stomach, and havc as good Effects on the Scurvy as the beft diftlilled Scurvy-Grafs , let it either be drawn off with Brandy, or of its felf.And alfo the Mornings draught the good Dame teaches her Hufband to drink , *(viz.)* Ale and Brandy mixed togerher,which will prove as beneficial. The like is to be underftood of other things called Medicines, if once the Multitude cries them up, tho they be never fo heterogcnc and improper, they muft do wonders, but leaving thcm to their own Humours, I fhall proceed to teach you feveral good Drinks againft the Stone and Gravel, and other Difeafes.

The beft Drinks to prevent the Generation, and Cure the Stone and Gravel, are fuch Drinks which God and his

Handmaid Nature have prepared to our hands, and is ready every where to be had (*viz.*) good River water; for the Stone and Gravel is hardly known in thoſe Countreys where the Natives common Drink is Water, for that of all others is the moſt friendly, mild, and cleanſing: But on the contrary, all firmented ſpirituous Drinks, let them be as wiſely handled as they can, neverthelefs they heat the Blood, and a little time does naturally cauſe them to tend towards heat, ſharpneſsſ and keneneſs,which qualities are great Enemies to the Human Nature and breaks the Harmony of the Humours, eſpecially in ſuch that are apt in Conſtitution to generate Gravel or the Stone; alſo ſulch Drinks cauſes the Diſtempers called Hcart-burnings, Fevers, and unnatural Heats throughout the whole Body; therefore ſuch as have a mind to preſerve their Healths, and be friends to their own Natures, let them follow theſe Directions, *viz.*

Of Cold Gruel.

TAke one ſpoonful of good Oatmeal, temper it with a little Water; then take a quart of the ſame cold Water,and brew the mixed Water and Oatmeal well together with the other quart, in two Pots that are for that purpoſe; and then it is done. Remember that your Oatmeal muſt be ground. The Oatmeal, if good, will mix or incorporate with the Water. Of this, ſort you may drink a pint or a quart, or more, at a time : This is a moſt excellent Drink to be drunk Mornings, and at Meals, or at any time of the day, and ſeaſon of the Year, for all ſorts of People, both for the healthy and unhealthy, eſpecially in hot Seaſons, and for ſuch who ate ſubject to the Stone, Gravel,or any other Obſtructions of the Paſſages; and for young People, the frequent and common uſe thereof does wonderfully ſtrengthen the whole Body, it is ſo friendly and homogeneeal, that it always quenches Thirſt the beſt of any others, by refreſhing the Spirits, bedewing the Body with a more pleaſant and more natural moiſture, than either Beer, Ale, Syder, or any other firmented Drinks. It begets a natural cheerfulneſs, extinguiſheth all kinds of natural Fluſhings and Vapors that comes for want of a ſtong, natural Health, and large Paſſageſs It opens and frees the Stomach and Paſſages from groſs Matter that obſtructs the digeſtive Faculties, and powerfully, purges by Urine, eſpecially if a quart or two be drunk in a Morning faſting. It.mightiy aſſiſts Nature in all her Operations, and it is not only profitable againſt the Stone and Gravel, but alſo gainſt gripling pains of the Bowles, helps Concoction, diſturbing the Stomach of ſuperfluous Juices, and cleanteth the Veſſels which are generally ſtopt and furr'd by Intemperance ; and it does naturally prevent Fumes and Vapor; by carrying the offending windy Matter into the Bowels, cauſing it to paſe with eaſe its proper way. Alſo the common uſe thereof excellent Remedy againſt ſhortneſs of Brcath, or other ill habits of the Stomach, and againdt all ſharp windy Humors and Juicus that falls into the Joins. And rica thing is a ſurcr and more powerfull Remedy againſt, the Scurvy and Dropſie, by oponing the Obſtructions of the Liver and Spleen begets *Appatite* to admiration; cheers and comforts the Spirits, and is in every reſpect friendly to Nature, and aſſiſt her in all her Operations. And whoſoever ſall accuſtom themſelves to the frequent drinking of this cold Gruel, ſhall find by experience greater benefit then I have here Set down. In all cold Seaſons you may warm your Water as you commonly do Ale or Beer, to that dcgree of heat which do rather better it then the contrary. It is alſo to be noted, that firm-entation, not only in Liquors, but alſo in Herbs and Vegitations, do deſtroy or tranſmute the opening mild friendly, cleanſ-ing and purging qualities, by Which they become of another nature and operation, for it changeth ſweetneſs into the higheſt degree of kenenefs and fharpnefs, opening the Body, and fee the Spints at liberty or on the wing, as is moft manifeft in Wort drawn from Mault, which is of an opening purging quality, but when firmented or workcd, and of ten or fourteen days old, fit to drink, then it is become another thing, for firmentation hath changed or tranfmuted thofe foft, mild, opening, friendly qualities into a brifk, lively, fpiritual Property, tending to heat, fharpnefs, and keenefs. The like is to be underftood in the Infufion of all opening Herbs in Wort, or the boyling them in Wort, and firmenting them afterward, therefore all forts of orening Liquors and Infufions are moft profitable againft the Stone, Gravel, and Obftruction of the Uritors before they be firmented of all, which our friendly cold Gruel hath the firft place ; but for fuch that have been accuftomed to Beer, Ale, Wine, and Syder, and are not willing to venter on our friendly Gruel, ought to drink all their firmented Liquors, new Ale a week, Beer twelve or fourteen days, and Syder and Wine new; and if they will uſe any opening Seeds or Herbs, then let them infuſe them in a pint of your Beer, Ale, Syder, or Wine one quarter of an hour before you drink, and warm it a little, ſo much as you do Ale or Beer when you drink it, which is a commendable way, far better then putting or infuſing the Herbs or Seeds in the Barrel, or working of them in the Wort. And you muſt remember that in all your infuſions that you uſe, infuſe but one Herb or Seed at a time, make no mixtures, leaſt inſtead of advancing, you quite deſtroy the natural and ſimple Operation of that from which you expect help, for few men do underſtand the genuine Nature and Operation of two or three ſeveal Herbs or Seeds, when mixed or infuſed together, much leſs when four, five, ſix, ſeven, eight, nine, ten, or twenty are jumbled together, as I have elſewhere demonſtrated.

Thoſe that deſire a morc friendly Ale then is generally drunk, may infuſe what quantity they pleaſe in there warm Wort, as you do Hops: Alſo uſe the Herb *Ale-hoof, Fennel Seeds, Caroways* and *Coriander,* all which are notable Purges by Urine; but they purge by Urine more powerful when infuſed in either new Ale or Becr, that is already firmented, as is mentioned before; ſo you may do; it in ſmall quantiyics, as you have occaſion: But if you infuſe thoſe, or any orher Herbs in Water, *(viz.)* in cold Water, for ten or twelve hours, and then drink a pint, or what you pleaſe; which have a far more powerful Operation againſt the fore-mentioned Diſtempers, then in any firmented Liquor. It is further to be conſidered, That ſtrong, ſtale, Beer, Syder, Wine, or any other firmented Liquors, the frequent drinking thereof do not only generate the Stone and Gravel, but they do as often occaſion the Gout, Conſumptions, Dropſies, and many other Diſeaſes, all according to the Nature of each mans Conſtitution, and what properly hath got the Aſcendant in the Humors of the Body, as is manifeſt in great Eaters and Drinkers ; one man drinks and eats himſelf into the Gout, another into a Conſumption, another into a Dropſie, or ſome other Diſtemper; the evil Effects are as various as their Natures and Conſtitutions are contrary. Be therefore reconciled to Water, that generous Element which without doubt was, and is the only Drink ordained for all Creatures by our Creator, therefore he that firſt firmented the Juices of the Grape, and made ſtrong Drink thereof, did drink and was drunk,and therefore was curſed with the greateſt of Curſes, which ought to be conſidered by all wiſe and good men; but Water is ſo friendly, and does contain many ſecret and admirable Virtues, which the Creator hath indued this Element with, as in all Ages hath been manifeſt; for it being pure and cleary in its own Nature; and is it not the only, and alone thing, by which all External things are purified, purged and cleanſcd? And though it be a vulgar Proverb, *As weak as Water;* yet I muſt tell you , Water is more ſtrong and ſublime then moſt imagine, for it contains a moſt raviſhing and excellent ſweet

Virtue, whence proceeds the pure, friendly, refreſhing quality,whereby it hath power, by its innate Virtue, to delight and purifie all ſorts of Food. Alſo in Preparations it is ſo innocent and friendly; that it diſſipates the groſsſ phlemy Body, and preſerves the more Eſſential Parts and Virtues, and keeps them living. What ſhall I ſay, words cannot declare its excellency; it is not only the moſt plentiful and truly pleaſant of all Drinks, but it ſupplies Nature with its friendly moiſture, and relieves Thirſt beyond all other Liquors or Juices, it is ſo ſimple, and indued with ſuch equality, that it inſinuates its mild opening Virtues into all parts of the Body in an inſenſible way; it makes no noiſe, nor cauſes any tumults in the Brain, nor awakens any inequality in the Body; but it imparts its meek Life as it were in ſilence ; and as Bread hath the firſt place of all Food, and mayjuſtly be called Concord, as being the foundation of all good Nouriſhment, the like is to be underſtood of Watcr, that being the Radix of all moiſt Nouriſhment, and renders all things fit and profitable for Mankind, of which there are great variety, all according to The Natures and Salniteral Virtues of the Earth it proceeds from; but for general uſe, Rain, River, and Spring-water are the beſt, and that of theſe ſorts that will waſh,brew,and perform all Preparations in Houſwifery is the beſt, *(viz.)* that Water that will waſh Lining to advantage is the beſt, which generally River-water will do, far better than moſt Springs, as I have demonſtrated in our *Way to Health.*

Cautions againſt certain Foods that Generate the Stone and Gravel.

FIRST, Such as are naturally ſubject to theſe Diſeaſes ought to refrain from all over-ſalt Fiſh and Fleſh; for ſuch things are not only hard of Concoction, furring the Paſſages, but they do heat the whole Body, and infect the Blood with a ſalt, ſharp, ſcorbutick Humour, occaſioning Crudities and evil Juices, obſtructing the Paſſages of the, whole Body, and eſpecially the Uriters.

Thirdly, Let them refrain all Spicy Foods, for they naturally heat the blood, hurt the natural heat, and produce the ſame Effects, eſpecially in youth.

Thirdly, Let them refrain all or moſt ſorts of Food made ſweet with Sugar, for the frequent uſe of ſuch Meats and Drinks do prove very prejudicial to moſt Peoples health, but more eſpecially to ſuch as are ſubject to the forementioned Diſeaſes ; for over-ſweetneſs in Foods and Drinks, does not only thicken the Blood, and hinder its free Circulation, but it indues it with a watery phlegmatick quality, and turns the Humours to the higheſt degree of ſouerneſs, more eſpecially if fats and ſweetneſs be compounded together, as they are for the moſt part (as the ſweeteſt Wines makes the ſharpeſt Vinegar) which immediately tends towards Putrifaction, whence proceeds various Difeafes, according to each mans Conftitution and Complexion, *viz.* fcabs, Boyls, Leprofies, Confumptions, Gout, and Stone, all Stoppages of the Breaft, ill Digeftion, Nautioufnefs, rotten Teeth, offenfive Breath, all which Diftempers have of late years been more brief and frequent, fince the common eating of fugered Foods and Drinks. And indeed moft Mothers and Nurfes, through an ignorant fond nefs, do lay the Foundations for thefe, and the like Difeafes in Children, from their very Infancy, by the continued ufe of fweetened Milks, and other compounded Foods; for Sugar, tho' it be the King of all Vegitations, and the fublimeft Salt the Vegitative Kingdom affords, as being more highly graduated in the almoft paradifical quality the Sweet; neverthelefs, that too frequent or over much eating of it proves baneful to Health; efpecially to young People and Children; for when it comes into the Stomach, and is there firmented, it prefently tends to kenenefs, fharpnefs, and fouernefs, which in many People proves of evil Confequence, and does generate a hard gretty Stone, making Subftance as it finds Matter capable, and difpofed to receive and joyn Forces with it.

Foyrthly, Alfo let thofe that are fubject to the forementioned Difeafes, forbear as much as in them lies, the frequent eating of fat fucculant Foods; for you muft note, that all fat Bodies are nothing fo eafily diffolvable, neither can the Natural *Minftrum* or Heat of the Stomach, fo well, digeft or make feparation thereof, as it can on Vegitation; neither do fuch things generate fo good Blood, or fine brifk lively Spirits; for this Caufe fat Foods lye long in the Stomach, and feem to fatiffie it, not that they afford more or better Nourifhment, but the reafon thereof is their oylinefs, as is manifeft in all External operations, for what *Menftrum* will eafily feparate and difoblve fat oyly things. The like is to be Underftood of the Stomach ; for this Caufe a man may eat double the quantity of lean Foods as he can of fat, and yet be more brifk, lightfom, and airy, and fooner an hungry again, efpecially when fed thereunto. Befides, fat Foods do not only fur the Paffages of the Uretors, and generate evil Juices there, but in all or moft phlegmetick conftitutions, obftructs the Stomach, caufing Coughs, and great increafe of Phegmatick Matter, whence grofnefs and fatnefs, fuch People does proceed; and the only and moft principal Foods to prevent fuch inconveniencs are fimple Vegitatons.

Fifthly, Improper Mixtures and Compofitions are to be avoided; as alfo baked, fryed, and ftewed Foods, and not to eat anything hotter than your Blood, and in Summer let all your Foods be quite cold, only fpoon Meats may be eaten as hot as Milk from the Cow; for whaffoever Food is taken hot, as the general Cuftom is, the fame is contrary to Nature, and does generate bad Blood, *viz.* makes it hot, fharp, and faltifh, which will manifeft it felf by breaking out in various Spots on the Flefh and Skin, commonly called *Symptoms of the Scurvy*; therefore confider the great and moſt wonderful work and myſtery of Nature in Generation ; and making of all Creatures, which is performed by a due hear and moiſture, the heat not exceeding that of our well tempered Blood, which we have treated on more fully in our *Way to Health.* The truth of theſe things, I think,, no wiſe man can deny, the ſame being ſenſibly demonſtrated by the Natives of thoſe Countreys, where they live for the moſt part on ſimple Foods, and innocent Drinks, viz. Water, which makes them ſtrangers to the Stone, Gout, Conſumption, and to many other Diſtempers that we are moſt generally afflicted with ; therefore those that would enjoy Healyh and long Life (which, amongſt all wiſe men, was, and is eſteemed a great bleſſing from the Lord) and prevent and cure themſelves of theſe Diſeaſes, let them; I ſay, apply themſelves to ſimple Meats, and ſuch Drinks as are before preſcribed, *viz.* to eat frely of Bread, Herbs, Gruels, boyl of Oatmeal and Wheat-flower, and all Foods made of Vegitations, which are of various ſorts, and yet natural and innocent, and every one may by practiſe learn how to apply them.

A good Drink againſt the Stone and other Stoppages.

TAke good Chalk, infuſe it in either River or Spring-water two, three, four, or ſix days, in open Veſſels in the Air, this is of excellent uſe, and very profitable againſt all ſtoppages and aſſid ſharp Juices that are ſubject to gripe the Stomach and Bowels; alſo it purges by Urine, and brings away Gravel and ſlimy offenſive Matter; for Chalk does naturally indue or impregnate the Water with a fine, mild, ſoft, friendly; or milky quality, very good againft Obſtructions and ſharp ſour Juices; it's taſte is pleaſant and grateful.

The good Houſwife may brew with this Chalky Water to great advantages for it makes excellent, mild, ſoft Ale, friendly to Nature. This Water alſo will waſh to great advantage, for it will ſave them both Labour and Soap. The truth is, Chalk is a brave, noble, Virgins Earth, of a Venerial Balſamic Natute and Operation, of admirable uſe and profit in the Manuring of all cold, ſtiff, claiey, Ground, it is to be preferred bcfore Lime,for one Manuring with Chaulk will continue its Virtues ſeveral years, but the Salniteral Virtue of Lime will not hold ſo long, becauſe in the burning of Lime the violent harſh fire of the Kill does totally deſtroy the mild, ſoft, friendly quality , and there does only remain the Original Salt, which is of an hot tart Nature and Operation, drying, and aſtringent; which qualities arc very profitable and uſeful in ſcvcral Trades and Arts, eſpecially in refning and making white Sugar, and indeed all ſorts of Sugar, it gives it Body and Life, cauſcs a

Coagulation.

But Chalk, being intire and ſimple, retains a moſt ſweet, allaying, mild, friendly Virtue, which alſo is one of the beſt things for Manuring Fruit-trees that ſtand in wet, cold Ground, to render them fruitful.

So Chalk being powdered, and put into Vinegar or Lime-Juice, it will preſently ſet it into a firmentation, and in a very little time it will allay or drink up the ſharpneſs or aſſidity thereof, ſo that it will become almoſt mild; alſo being put into the fierce, corroding, keen Spirit of Salt, it will in ſome meaſure. allay, its fiery ſharpneſs. Likewiſe, if the powder of Chalk be put into hard ſtale Beer, Syder, or Mum, and ſtir or brew it together, and then let it ſtand two or three minutes, and it will preſently ſettle; it will drink new, mild and pleaſant, and alſo very wholſom and palatable, ſo wonderful is its qualifying, friendly, mild nature, and without doubt it does contain many great Secrets (the diſcovcring of which is not ſitable to this place) what is ſaid being ſufficient to inſinuate the uſefulneſs thereof both in Huſbandry aud Houſewifery,and Phyſick, in which laſt Reſpect, for the preſervation of Health, I recommend it to all People, eſpecially to thoſe that are ſubject by Nature or Accident to thoſe terrible Diſtempers the Stone and Gout. Furthermore, 'tis a common Experiment when People are troubled with the Diſtemper, vulgarly called Heart-burnt, to beat or powder a little Chaulk, and put it to Water and drink it, which gives them eaſe; but the reaſon of the Cure few conſiders. I conceive that that Diſtemper does not ſo pro- perly afflict the Heart, as reſides about the Orifice of the Stomach, ariſing from a ſharp, keen, ſour, burning Humor or Firment, occaſioned by Exceſs and ill Digeſtion, which ſeems to inflame thoſe Parts; now the drinking of Water, in which Chalk is infuſed, does by its mild Balſamick Virtues, allay or mitigate that ſhort ſevereneſs or violence, and thereby gives the Party eaſe; for if is hath ſuch a power when only outwardly infuſed in ſtale

Beer, Syder, Mum, Wine, of Vinegar and other eager Liquors, 'tis but reaſonable to believe it will have no leſs ſignal Operation, when taken in a proper quantity inwardly, where the friendly powers of Nature are ready to aſſiſt, and help advance to the higheſt Mergie, for removing and ſubduing thac which before afflicted and oppreſſed them.

A good and profitable way for the Poor, and wholſom for the Rich, to make Cherry wine, or Drink of Gooſberries, Currans, Apricocks and Plumbs, being eaſie and wholſom, pleaſant and cheap. There being but one way and manner in the making and operation, therefore one Example will ſerve for all.

TAke ripe Cherries, Gooſe-berries, Plumbs, Currans, or any of the like Fruits, bruiſe them in a convenient veſſel, then put them in a Tub, ſuch as a one as you maſh your Mault in when you brew, with a Tap in it, then put what quantity of good water (*viz.* cold) as you pleaſe, as you would have your Drink, ſmall or ſtrong; let theſe Cherries infuſe twelve, fourteen, ſixteen, or eighteen hours, then draw it off, and if it be to keep infuſe ſome bitter Herbs or Seeds in it three hours; but if it be for preſent drinking then *Balm*, or any other good Herb: After this, add to every Gallon two or three pound of Treakle, or two or three pound of Sugar or Hony, but if you would have it very ſtong, then add more ſweetning; then take ſome Yeſt or Barm, and put it a Working, as you do Beer or Ale. The ſame method you may obſerve in all orher Fruits, as Gooſberries, Currans, and the like. This ſort off Drink or Wine is to be preſented before that which is made of the whoIe Juice, eſpecially if your Sugar be good; it drinks finer. and lighter on the Stomach, andmore warm, not ſo apt to ſend fumes into the Head, and will digeſt any ſort of Food much better than that which is commonly made.

There is another way of ma king this ſort of Drink,(*viz.*)Take good Water, and make it ſcalding hot, put it into your Maſh-tub to your bruiſed Fruits, and let them infuſe one hour, then draw it off infuſe your Herbs or Seeds in it, if they be bitter half an hour, if not, then an hour, then put it a cooling as you do Wort, and then put your Sugar, Treakle, or Hony, what, quantity you think fit, or as you would have it in ſtrength, then add ſome Yeſt, ſrir it well together, and it will firment or work, and ſo barrel it; but cold Water from the Fountain iſ to be preferred before hot, and is much a briſker Wine.

Theſe are eaſie,cheap, familiar and makes woſt excellcnt Drink. If your Fruits be of your own Growth, it will then ſtand you but in a ſmall martcr, very little more than ordinary Beer,and be much ſtronger. This ſort of Drink every poor man may have; and indeed it is a better, and more wholſomer Drink or Wine then the common ſort made by preſſing; for Water is the Homogenial *Menſtrum* in the World, and moſt familiar to Human Nature; and by this way of Operation, it mildly and ſweetly draws forth all the good Virtus of the Fruit without force and violence and leaves the harſh, bitter aſtringency of the Stones and Skins behind, whereas preſſing doth by its violence force forth the bitter harſhneſs both of the Stones and Skins, and is very hurtful, as is clearly ſeen in Syder and Wine, for the Stones and Skins are of a harſh, bitter aſtringent Nature and Operation; for hard bruiſing, and violent preſſng of tender Fruits, do not only extract and force forth the harſhneſs of the Stones and Skins, but it does as it were ſuffogate or diſmay the fine, lively, ſpirituous qualities, which your Senſe of Taſting will tell you. Taſte the Fruit before it be bruiſed or preſſed, and then the Juice, that proceedeth from them,the Juice drawn out by our mouth, is fine, briſk, and penetrating ; but the Juices preſſed out are dull, heavy, and groſs to thc Palate and Stomach. The ſame is manifeſt in the Juices prcſſed out of green Hcrbs; for Example, Take what ſort, or ſorts, of Sallad Herbs, bruiſc them to maſh, then take them and diſh them into a Sallad, and they will be ſo groſs, dull, heavy, and fulſom, to both Pailate and Stomach; but thoſe ſame Herbs that are diſhcd up into a Sallad, which are not bruiſed will be moiſt, pleaſant, and grateful. Now hcrc you ſee that this hard. bruiſing and preſſng, hath as it were wholly deſtroyed the briſk lively Virtues, and indeed all that is deſirable or delightful both to the Senſes, as well as to the Stomach.

Note that the forementioned Drinks that are made of Water, Herbs, Fruit, Sugar, Treakie, or Hony, are beſt with cold Water, as I have told you before eſpecially in hot Countries, for fiered Drinks are no friends to Nature, except wiſely handled; rherefore the Natives of those Climates, where they drink Water, are not known to have the Stone, and where their Foods are ſimple, which-all wiſe men ought to conſider.

Laſtly, Note that all ſorts of Syder would keep much better, and be far wholſomer, eſpecially for ancient People, and ſuch are more or leſs ſubject to the Stone or Gravel, if when it is new made you infuſed in part of it, bitter Herbs, gathered and prepared as we

have taught in our *Way to Health, viz. Wormwood, Hops, Cardis Century, Sage, Betiny, Dandelion* or the like, for the bitter quality does naturally hold the ſweet Body and Volatile Spirits, as it were, captive, for *Mars* loves *Venus,* alſo bitterneſs does mightily withſtand and moderate the keen, aſtrigent, hard, harſh propertics; that they cannot advance nor devour the ſweet, mild qualities; for this cauſe all bittet Herbs dopreſerve all ſorts of Drinkſ, and keep them from ſharp hardneſs and aſtringency, longer then otherwiſe they would. Beſides,they are wholſom, pleaſant, and healthful when People are uſed to
them.

Alſo good ſtore of ſuch Herbs, whoſe predominant quality ſtands in bitterneſs, ought to be infuſed in all Drinks made of Sugar, Mallyſ, Treakle, or Hony, becauſe ſuch Liquors or Drinks tends to a ſharp keneneſs ſooner then Drinks made of Mault, which our Engliſh and others, ought to conſider that inhabits, the *Weſt-Indies,* and other hot Climates, where they frequently make various ſorts of Drinks with Sugar, MaIlas, and Fruits, and where alſo they are terribly afflicted with the Stone, Gout, and Gravel, *viz.* which all or moſt Drinks made of Sugar or MaIlas are apt to generate; for the higheſt Sweets, when firmented, either in Liquors, or in the Stomach, quickly tends to the higheſt ſharpneſs and keen harſhneſs, eſpecially in ſome Conſtitutions, if the ſweet quality be not ſome degrees alaid or captivated by the bitter, which do alſo moderate or withſtand the aſtringent band.

Having had Experience and certain Know- ledge of the Virtues of theſe Preparations,
I thought it my Duty to Communicate to the World, for the benefit of ſuch as ſhall pleaſe to make uſe of them, and for ſuch as ſcorn and deride them, they ſhall, though they ſlight- my poor Advice, injoy my Cordial, Pity.

AN

APPENDIX

SHEWING

The Natural Caufes why Fruit-Trees do fo frequently fail Bearing, and Offering Expediments to make Orchards almoft conftantly frnitfiul. With a new Experiment of preferving of Eggs fweet and good for feveral Months.

HAving in our other Writings occafionally difcourfed of Syder, and how advantagioufly the fame might be made, efpecially to Farmers and poor Country People, I fhall here take leave to add a few Confiderarions touching Fruit-Trees.

Tis certain, that planting of Orchards, as it is a thing of great Delight, and but of little Labour, and that moſt Natural and Agree-able unto the firſt Commandment of our Creator, ſo it might be as Profitable an Imployment of Ground as any whatſoever. The only thing, I conceive, that diſ eourages many People, is, That Fruit-Trees, eſ-pecially old planted, ſeldom brings any conſiderable Crop; for if they bear full one year, its odds but the next they miſs, nay often till the third and fourth year after, they yield not any conſiderable quantity of Fruit, the Reaſon of which is commonly attributed to great Froſs, ſharp Winds, uncouth Seaſons, Blaſts, and Blithes from unwholſom Air, and ſuch like Eternal Accidents. But I conceive the true Reaſon is more natural, conſtant, and ſettled, and being once known, might without much difficulty be remedied from things known, we by an equality of Reaſon, may probably gueſs at like things, tho' unknown. Now methinks, in the Huſbandry of Corn, we have every day Inſtances, very probable to this of Trees, only what is conſtantly practiſed in one Caſe, iſ not regarded in the other.

It is Rule in Huſbandry, not to ſow one ſort of Grain or Corn two, three, or four years on one piece of Ground. For Example, Break up Ground, if it be good; ſtrong, loomy Earth, they, will ſow Beans; if weakcr or light, Oats; after the Beans or Oats, Wheat; after Wheat, Barly; after Barly, peas or Rye. But if the hand be dunged every year, or every other year, then you may ſow Barly or Wheat,Beans or Peas two years together; becauſe the freſh dunging of it does add or ſtrengthen the Salniteral Properties or Virtues, which was much ſpent or wcakned, or drawn forth by the former years Crop. Nor does any diſcrcet Huſbandman expect a good Crop of any Grain, if he ſows it ſeveral years together on the ſame Field, except he dung it; nor will that do, if he perſiſt in ſowing one and the ſame ſort two, three, or four years one aftcr another; for the Dung cannot rcpleniſh ſuch Land eith a ſufficient quanity of that Natural Salniteral Virtue, Fat, or Juices that is proper for the Nouriſhment and Augmentation of the ſame kind of Grain ſo often repeated.

Thus tis plain that each ſort of Grain (and conſequently every, other Vegitation, of what Species ſoever it bc) does by Simile, attract and draw unto its ſelf, out of the Bowels of the adjacent Ground wherein they grow, ſuch a particular Nutrative Virtue or Juice, as is proper and natural for the Nouriſhment and Propagation of its own Body: And tho' every ſort of Corn,and other things, has, and is indued with all the ſevenfold Forms and Properties of Naturc, yet in each thing there iſ ſome one quality or property that is chief, or moſt predominant, and which does draw from the Earth what is agreeable to its ſelf, and ſo leaves the contigious Ground barren or poor, as to the particular Juice , tho' yet ſtill by a general Salniteral fatneſs, may be in very good heart, ſtrong and apt to produce Vegitations of another kind, if one and the ſame Corn be continued, it will prove thin poor, weak, and dwindling, anſwering neither the Hope nor Charge and Toyl of the Huſbandman, but if another Corn (tho' ſuch as naturally requircs a richer Mould then the other) be ſowed there, it ſhall flouriſh; nay, tho' yon dung your Land frequently, yet if you ſow the ſame Grain more than one yea r,if the Seaſon prove not extream kind, ſuch Corn will be apt to fail, and come to little, as often happens near *London,* where they dung their Ground much, becauſe they till it every year, and many times twice a year: So that if Huſbandmen ſhould continue one ſort of Grain for ſeveral years together on the ſame Land, there would be as great, or greater Scarcity and Want of Corn, as there happens to be of Apples and other Fruits.

For what we have obſerved in ihe Tilling and Manuring Land for Corn, and the method of making the Ground conſtantly fruitful, by changing the Species of the Grain committed to it, holds good (as to the former part) in all kind of Fruit-Trees, but the ſame method (as to the latter part) for the Remedy cannot be obſerved in the management of them, as in Land for Corn, and therefore they often miſs, and much the oftner for not being ſo well ordered and manured as they might, and ought to be. In Huſbandry you change your Grain, and often dung your Land,whereby it is in ſome meaſure furniſht with a Recruit of every ſort of Juice; but Trees cannot be every year or two tranſ-planted out of one Ground into another, nay, ſcarce at all when they grow big, but are commonly continued thirty, forty, or ſixty years, or more, in the ſelf ſame Place or Ground. Now Trees being generally planted near together (which by the way is a very great Error in planting of Orchards, robbing each other, not only of nouriſhment from above) and being of great Bulk and Subſtance, large Roots and ſpreading Branches, they muſt needs require great ſtore and quantity of Nouriſhment to ſupport their Life, Growth and Fruit, even much more then moſt ſorts of Earth can adminiſter, for every Tree doth powerfully draw forth of the Earth ſuch a Salniteral Virtue or Juice, as is proper to Maintain and Nouriſh its own Body, which no Earth can continually afford, except it be much helped by Art; for as wc have ſhewed in the Management of Land for Corn, ſo the Ground, where Fruit-Trees grow, will in proceedſ of time become poor, ſour, and hungry, as to the Virtue that is proper for the Nouriſhment and Support of Trees, and thercfore they are not able to bring forth or bear Fruit every year. The very ſame inconveniences would happen to Corn, if the Land were not often dunged, limed, or the like, and the, Grain changed frequently ; therefore the principal Cauſe why Fruit-Trees do ſo often blight, or miſs bearing, is not ſo much from External cold ſharp Airs (tho' they may ſometimes do miſchief, or at leaſt help forward the evil) as Internally, for want of ſufficicient Nouriſhment; for if Land cannot bring forth good Crops for ſeveral years, one after another, of the ſame Corn, (which is inconſiderable, as to Subſtance and Bulk, in reſpect of Fruit-Trees) how then can it be cxpected that an Orchard ſhould bear plentifully every year, where there is neither Change, nor Tillage, nor Dunging, it may be for the ſpaceof thirty or forty years; and many times, the Trees planted too thick, that the Sun Beams can hardly Influence the Earth. 'Tis true, ſome Trees will bear every year, others every other, and ſome every third year, according to the Nature of the Earth and Fruit, for that year or two that they bear not, is as it were a Sabbath unto the Earth and Trees; or like Land whcn it lies fallow in which time they get heat, and repleniſh themſelves with ſtrength and virtue, which inward virtue does withſtand all ſharp and pinching keen Airs, that they hurt not; for if the Internal Salniteral Virtue or Radical Moiſture be ſtrong, whence all Vegitations hath its vigorous Birth, then there is little or no danger of Outward Acci- dents ; but on the contrary, when the Inward Oyl and

Nourifhing Juices are weak and impotent, then every Outward fmall Accident, as Frofts, cold fharp Winds, and the like, do take place, and help forward the Evil. The like is to be underftood in the Human Nature, and Animal Kingdom: If a man be of a crafie, impotent Conftitution or Nature , then every cold Air or little Accident will wound his Health; or if any particular Member or Limb be weakned or difordered, that fame Part, upon any Outward Heat or Cold, or other Accident,will fuck in the Injury, and beafily made more weak and impotent; which does hold good in all things, whether Vegitations or Animals, according to the Nature of each; for this Gaufe it often happens when we have very warm, mild Springs, little or no Frofts, or fharp Eafterly winds, (which of all are efteemed the moft pernicious to fruit) that there is but little Fruit the following Summer: On the contrary, other years, when there happens cold North, and North-Eaft wind and fevere Frofts, great ftorc of moft forts of Fruits, the truth of this every Country man does know; and yet for all this, all their cry is, All our Fruit is blaſted in one froſty cold Night, or a ſharp Wind, never ſo much as conſidering, that other years they have had great ſtore of all ſorts of Fruit and yet far colder and ſharper Springs; but moſt People do in this, as they do by themſelves, every Diſorder that happens to them, they attribute to outward Cold and Accident that comes that way, and hardly think of the inward Cauſes, Intemperances and other Violences they offer to Nature, whence moſt or all Obſtructions does ariſe and proceed, as we have largely demonſtrated in our other Writings.

The truth of what we have before declared, is further manifeſted by this, *viz,* if you cut down an old Orchard, and cleanſe the Ground as well as you can from the Roots, and then plant young Trees in the old ones places, neither the one nor the other will thrive, nor come to any Maturity, but are very Scrubs, and often dye, and come to nothing, at leaſt not thrive, or grow ſo much in ten years as thoſe in new Ground will in three or four; the chief Reaſon thereof is, becauſe the Ground in which old Orchards ſtood, is as it were deſtitute of, or contain very little of that Radical Juices or Salniteral Virtues, that is proper for the Nouriſhment of ſuch Fruit-Trees (ſince the foregoing Trees) but all new ground, eſpecially ſuch as is proper for Fruit-Trees, does abound, and is impregnated with that Salniteral Juice and Virtue, as is clear by thriving and proving of Trees there planted. Moreover, moſt or all old Orchards, the Boughs, Limbs, and Branches of the Trees are covered with a certain Moſs, of a dry, huſky, harſh, aſtringent Subſtance, which does ariſe for want of a proper quantity of Nouriſhment, that ſtops the Paſſages and Pores, hindering the true Circulation of the Radical Moiſture, and then the Eſſential Juices becomes tough, and as it were ſtagnated, which preſently deſtroys the lively Complexion and Beauty of that thing; and when ſoever this happens in

Trees, presently a mossy Scurfgrows on the Limbs and Boughs, like unto Scurf or a mangy Disease in Animals; for when the Ground, by the long standing of Trees, grows poor, hungry, and barren, as to the virtue that Treesh delight in, then that Nourifhmcnt that they do draw forth is not good, neither doth it generate good Juices, and the Trecs begins to Languish and bccomc Consumptive, which is the true Cause of Moss, Cankers, Blithes, and the like; and yet that same Ground, if Manured for other things, as Beans , Peas, and thc like will bear great Crops, for it was rich enough in that Salniteral quality that wasproper and natural for the Nourishment of such Grain, but poor and out of heart in respect of Trees, but if you cut down an old Orchard, and Manure the Ground for Various sorts of Corn, and Dung it as other Land for eight or twelve years (the longer the better) then plant a young Orchard, the Trees will thrive pretty well, for in this time the Earth hath recovered and strengthened the weakened fading Salnitenal virtues proper for Trees, but not ſo ſtrong and vigorous as that Ground that never had Fruit-Trees planted in it. But here ſome will Object, Why ſhould not Fruit-Trees thrive and bear without manuring and dunging, as well as other Trees, *viz.* Oaks, Elms, Hazels, and the like, which will grow in one ſort of Ground without any dunging or manuring for many ſcore years. I Anſwer; Tis to bc underſtood that all ſuch Ground in which Oaks, Hazels, and the like, grow, is principally indued with ſuch a quality as is proper to bring forth and nouriſh ſuch Trees, and conſiſts chiefly thereof, and therefore ſuch Woods will grow naturally there without planting, as well as without manuring. So all good Ground will bring forth Graſs, more or leſs, as the Seaſon is kind, or on the contrary. But our Apples, Pears, andmoſt ſorts of Wall-fruit, does not ſo naturally grow in our Climate, any more then ſeveral ſorts of our Garden Herbs, which, both Trees and Herbs, are all managed by Art, and great Induſtry, or elſe they will dwindle away and come to nothing, tho' Field Herbs are plenty enough naturally, ſo that every thing muſt be managed according to its kind, and there iſ no parity between Fruit-Trees and other common Trees, both for theReaſon juſt now given, as eſpecially becauſe the latter does not bare any Annual Crop as the former, but if the Trunk and Branches live and grow it's enough, whereas you expect much more from your Orchards, and therefore muſt be at more pains with it. Sometimes you ſhall ſee in the Spring aTree bravely bloſſomed, and yet at *Autumn* no Fruit; the Reaſon is commonly aſcribcd to Blaſting or Froſts; but I believe it may moſt times be referred to the Cauſe before mentioned; for in the early Spring the Sun giving every thiig vigor, the Soyl made ſhift to ſupply the Tree with Radical Moiſture enough to make that ſhow, but not being able to continue its Recruits, the poot Tree could not perform its Promiſe, nor Nature accompliſh its Intentions. But you'l ſay, What Remedy for all this? Can you ſhew a

Natural way to keep and tender Trees capable of bearing every year, or for the moſt part. I Anſwer you, and it is thus: Digg three, four, five, or ſix yards about each Tree, to, the Root, carry away moſt of the Earth, and ſupply the place with freſh Earth mixed with a little Dung, alike quantity to which you carried away, and this you ought to do every three, four, ot five years, or as often as the Farmer dungs his Land for Corn, which will give ſuch Life, Power, and Virtue to your Trees, that you need not much doubt of a Crop every year, or at leaſtwiſe it will ſeldom miſs, and your Fruit will be large and fair; but if thiſ be too much trouble and charge; then digg or trench your Orchard, and Dung it well once in two,three, or four years, which may ſerve indifferent well. The very ſame management ought to be obſerved in all ſorts of Wall-Fruit-Trees, and others. It is alſo to be noted, That when you plant Orchards or Walls in poor, hungry Gravel or hot Sandy Ground, then you ought to Trench your Ground very deep, and at the bottom to lay ſtore of good black Mould, or Earth mixed with Dung, and then turn in the upermoſt or ſurface of the Earth, and carry away the upermoſt Gravel or Stoney Earth, for that is ſo hungry, hot, and lean, that if it be mixed with the good Earth, it will as it were, eat out or deſwtroy the good Virtues thereof; but if you will not be at the trouble and charge of digging up and trenching all your Ground, then digg large Holes, and carry away theuppermoſt Gravel, Sand, or Clay, and ſupplythe place with good Earth, or Dung and Earth mixed together, and then plant your Tree in it a proper depth, *viz.* ſo deep as your Tree did naturally grow, for deeper is injurious to the Plant; and when you have filled your.Earh in about your Tree , within a little, then put a little good Dung around your Tree near the Surface, and cover it with Earth, which will keep the Roots of your Tree cool in Summer, and warn in the Winter.

It is alſo to be notcd, That if your Ground be hot and ſandy, then mix or manure your

Trees with good Loom, Dung, and black Earth; if gravelly, hungry ground, then good Mold and Dung mixed together; if cold clayte Ground, then mix Chalk and Earth together; which, if this Order be obferved, it will mightily advance and caufe your Trecs, not only to thrive, but bear more and larger Fruit. It is alfoto be noted, That the old Cuftom of opening the Earth; and laying bear the Roots of Fruit Trees in the Winter Seafon, is an Error in Hufbandry, except there be immediately the old Earth taken away, and the place thereof fupplied with good frefh Earth, or Earth amd Dung weII mixed, fuch as Trees have never grown in, as is mentioned before, for that Earth that covers the Roots are their natural Cloathing, which do fecure them from the Injury of the Element, keeping them warm in the Winter, and cool and moisft in the Summer, the Earth being many Degrees warmer in the Winter then the common Air, but in the Summer as many cooler; therefore the uncovering of the Roots, and expofing them for two or three

Months to the cold pinching Airs, *viz.* Froſt, Snow, Rains, and violent Winds, muſt needs be unnatural, and conſequently prove prejudicial by weakning the inward Power and Salniteral Virtues of ſuch Trees, rendring them the more uncapable of bearing the following Summer. Conſult Nature, and ſhe will teach you the Truth of what we have here declared. Will not all Gardeners, when they dig up a ſmall Tree, as Gooſberries, Currants, and the like, if they cannot conveniently plant them preſently, cover the Root in Earth ſo deep as they naturally grow, which are inconſiderable Trees in compariſon of large Fruit-Trees, and moſt of them will as naturally grow as weeds.

Note, That the moſt natural and proper time for planting moſt or all Fruit-Trees, is from the middle of *October* to the laſt of *December*, for by early planting the Earth and the Roots do not only ſettle well together, and unite, but the Roots do draw and grow, and thereby they are not only more forward then late planted Trees, but alſo they will the better indure any hot, dry Seaſon that may happen the following Summer. The ſame Time or Seaſon is to be obſerved in pruning and cutting ſuperflous Branches, the earlier in the year it is done the better; for every Branch or Limb that is Cut off from the Body is a certain Wound, and the Tree cannot recover that Injury till it haſ paſſed a Spring and Summer; the Truth of this is demon- ſtrated by their not bearmg ſo plentifully the fellowing Summer ; therefore the earlier they are pruned, the more time they have to recover ſuch Inconveniences ; and if you do Cut off any eminent Limb or Branch, then you ought to take the ſame Compoſition of Earth you uſe in grafting, which is generally done with good Loomy Earth, mixed with a little Cow-dung tempered well, then cover or plaiſter the cut Limb or Branch, which will keep the Wound or Place warm, and heal and preſerve it from the drujury of a ſevere Winter, as cold, ſharp, pinching Airs, Froſts and Winds, penetrating Rottenneſs and

Ranknefs and other Diftempers that often happens to fuch wounded Parts. The like is to be underftood of the laying of the Rots of Trees open, as is mentioned bcfore, and expofing them bare faced to a fevere Winter, and Injury of the Elements, as extream Cold, Wet and Winds, for under the Surface of the Earth the Natural heat is not only greater and ftronger, but more conftant than the common Air in Winter Seafons, which is varied and changed according as the Eye of the World increafes or decreafes, and from what quarter of the Heavens the Wind blows; which is further manifefted by moft or all fountains and Springs, which in Summer or hot Seafons, the Waters proceeding out of the Earch,at the Head thereof are many degrees colder then the common Air; or the Waters of other Rivers that runs on the Surface of the Earth; but in Winter, or in cold Seafons, at the Head of the fame Springs or Fountains, the Water thereof is as many degrees warmer then either the common Air, or the Waters of Rivers that runs on the

Source of the Earth; for this caufe, in cold Seafons or in Winter, we can fee them fend forth Fumef and Vapors, which is chiefly occafioned by the Conttrarieties the two, Qualities, *viz.* Heat and Cold ; not but all or moft Fountaing, Springs, Rivers, and other Waters, and alfo the whole Earth, do continually and at all times, more or lefs, breathe forth Fumes and Vapors, the degree thereof is according to the Nature and Conftitution of the Elements, Seafon of the Years and Celeftial Influences though these Vapors and Fumes which the Sun and Celeftial Bodies do continually exhale, cannot be feen but only when the Air is colder than the Earth, which cold keen Air does immediately condenfe thofe Vapors, that they become viffible; but when the Earth and Air are of an equal Temperture, then you cannot fee thofe Fumes no more than you can fee your own breath in a wart Seafon ; but you muft not conclued that you do not breath becaufe you do fee it: and it is as natural for the Earth and Water to breathe and ſend forth Fumes and Vapors as for Animals, and they do ariſe and proceed from the Central life of the Elements, for without Motion nothing could ſubſiſt neither cauld the Earth, Waters, or any of the Elements generate or bring forth any living Creature, if they had not thiſ natural Motion, there being a continual ſympathetical Operation and Mixion of all Qualities, and Elemants, But it is to be noted, that ſome ſorts of Grounds and Waters, and alſo in ſome Seaſons of the Year, thoſe Fumes and Vapors are more plentifuuly lent forth then in order; as after an hot Summer, in *Auguſt*, *September*, and *October* the Elemnents then being morſt and and full of Humidity, occaſioned by the Declination of the Sun, the Days warm, the Nights cold, which do condenſe thoſe warm Vapors that the Earth and Waters breathes and ſends forth. Now theſe Streams or Breathes, which are nothing elſe but the natural Motions of innate Life and Operations of Nature; are better or worſt, good, or bad, healthy or unhealthy; according to the

Nature and quality of the Waters, and ſituation of thc Ground, which they proceed from. Now theſe Steems or Vapors that ariſes and proceeds from clear Founains and Springs, or from running Rivers eſpecially ſuch as have Flux and Reflux, as the River of Thames, and many others have, are fine, moiſt, thin, and penetrating, and are powerful openers of Obſtructios, and great Preſervers of Na ture, and begets Appetite, and are good againſt Aſtmatical Diſtempers of the Breaſt, eſpecially if the quality and quantity of Meats and Drinks be carefully obſerved; but the contrary is to be underſtood of thoſe Steems and Vapors that ariſes and proceeds from low boggy Grounds, Pools, ſtanding Waters, and the like, which do agree but with few Conſtitutions, except ſuch as are born and bred in ſuch places; and tho good Airs are great Preſervers of Health, yet Temperance and Order hath the firſt place, and ought to be regarded above all other Circumſtances, and if that be wanting, Other things and obſervations ſignifies little.

It is alſo to be noted, That all Waters do more plentifully breathe forth Steems and Vapors than the Earth, as being more penetrable, thin, and tranſparent, and therefore more capable of receiving the Light and ſſweet Inflences of the Celeſtrial than the Earth, which is a cloſe, firm, compacted, dark Body in compariſon, of the Element of Water; therefore the Vapors proceeding from the Earth are heavier, duller, and fewer in quantity, but not ſo thin, nor penetrating in quality as theſe from the Water; for this Cauſe thoſe Perſons,whoſe Imployments are in and about Waters, have for the moſt part greater Appetites than others, and are more lively, briſk and ſtrong. Therefore it is very good for all People that are afflicted with ſhortneſs of Breath, Stoppages at the Stomach, or overfatneſs, to imploy thenſelves on Waters, or uſe themſelves to walk to by Rivers ſides, as much as they can, in all Seaſons of the Year; but morc eſpecially in Spring and Summer; for thoſe fine, thin cool, penetrating Vapors, are as it were ſuckt in on all ſides of the Body, which do render thoſe, whoſe. Imployments are abroad; briſk, lively, and healthful, more eſpecially in moderate Seaſons and when the Air and Elements are a little inclinable to Humidity which do mightily rarifie the Air and make it more penetrating; and all Men and Beaſt are not ſo ſubject to heat and drought, and other Indiſpoſitions, as in hot, dry Seaſons ; for heat and drought do not only, as it Were, cloſe up the Poors of the Earth, but it thickens and ſtagnates the Air, conſuming the fine thin, moiſt penetrating Vapors and Spirits, making them thick , hot, and ſulpherous, and hinders the natural Motions and Circulations of the Elements, and their Salniteral Virtues. Now this Motion, Circulation, and continual Sympathatical Mixtion of the Elements, is further mani-feſted by the Sea, which is the Center of the Element of Water, the Moon being the Governeſs thereof, the having a certain, ſecret Influence according to her Increaſe,

Decreaſe, and Configurations ſhe hath with the Celeſtial Bodies; for if there were not a continual Motion in this great Fountain, Tides, Flux and Reflux , there could be no Creatrure generated; or ſhould there be a Ceſtation from Motion but a few hours, the whole would immediately become a ſtinking Lake and all her Inhabitants would be deſtroyed; for that which we call Tides , is nothing but the natural Motion and Circulation that proceeds from the Center or Heart, and Animals can as well ſubſiſt and cotinue there, being without Motion and Circulation of the Blood, and breating as the great Fountains of Waters or other Elements can live or give being to their Children, without Motion and continual Circulation, which ariſes and proceeds from an innate power of the Elements; for theſe Elements are the great Body and wonderful Powers of God, and by his centeral Word and innate Virtue, all things, both in the Animal, Vegitable,and Mineral Kingdoms, have been,and are made, generated, and preſerved;

for the whole Globe of Earth, Water, Fire and are the living Powers of God, in which his holy W ord do continually create and bring to, manifeſtation the hidden Myſteries and Wonders both of Time and Eternity, to his eternal Praiſe and Glory, and his Work goes alway on in exact Number, Weight and Meaſure, for in God, nor in his Handmaid Nature, there is no ſuch thing as ſtanding ſtill or idlneſs; for ſhould the *Primum Mobile* ceaſe from its natural Motion and Circulat-ion, but a few Minutes, the whole *Mundam Siſtime* would be ready to ſink into Confuſion; for ſtanding ſtill, or idleneſs, have no ſympathy either with God or Nature ; for the Heaven, Stars, and Elements, with the wonderful and amazing Varieties of Beaſs, Fiſhes, Vegitation and Minerals, wherewith the lower 'Worlds are indued and furniſhed, are the living Powers and Works of the Lord, and are ſtill continued by his Alwiſe Providence and Divine Word, which is never idle; for Idleneſs, as is ſaid before, is allowed no being, either in the Internal or External

Worlds ; all in the Bcginning was brought into a Being through Labour and Motion, as the Learned *Moſes* faith *The Lord moved himſelf on the face of the Waters,* and they are utill ſuſtained to this day by the ſame active and working Power of the Creator Confider the daily Motions and Circulations of the Celeſtials, *viz.* Sun, Moon, and wonderful Company of Stars, their Riſing, Setting, continual Motion, Courſes, and various configurations, and all in exact Order: Behold the Fountains, Springs, and Rivers labouring continually in a long progreſs to pay their tributary Streams to the Ocean and the Ocean by induſtrious Tides, FIux and Refluxes, ſtriving as it were to ſupply the Land from its innate or central Power. Do not the great Eye of the World by a ſympathaticatcal Power and univerſal Motion of all Elements, exhale Moyſture from the Fountains of Waters, and bottle it up in the Clouds or Powers of God till an appointed time, and then Rcturn it with plenteous Uſury, to water and make fat the

Earth with the Dew of Heaven? And are not the like Circular Motions and variety of Powers underſtood in Man? And is not he a little World out of the great? In him is contained the true Nature and Operation of all Elements; and yet, what great Matters can he do or perorm without Motion and Acton? Are not all theſe neceſſary things, that ſervcs for the ſupport and accommodation of Human Life, are not, nor cannot be procured without Labour and Motion? Nay, Life it ſelf cannot otherwiſe be maintained,the Blood muſt always be circulating, the Pulſe Natures Clock, continually ſtriking, the Stomach muſt labour hard in her Kitchin to dreſs, and prepare, and ſeparate Aliment; for the other Parts, the Lungs be buſie in Tranſpiration, the Heart ſending forth Reſerves and new Supplies of Spirits to all the Frontier Gariſons and riemote Limbs of the Body, whilſt the Brain is no leſs ſolictiouſ to give the neeſſary Orders from the Grand Councel, held, between, the Underſtanding, the Will, and the Judgment, whereunto Inteligence every Minute arrives from the five Sally Ports, called the Senſes, and all their Reſults are carefully Regiſtred, and treaſured up by the Recorder, Memory; nay, ſhould the hands grow ſlugiſh, and neglect the ſupplying the Stomach' with Food, the Mouth would ſoot be open to upbraid their Lazineſs; from all which, tis a parent, as if written with the Sun-beams, that ſtanding ſtill or idleneſs hath no Being in God, nor in Works, but all the Elements, and other numerous Off-ſprings, do labour with higheſt Diligence for to manifeſt the wonderful Myſteries of their Beings, which all Mankind ought ſeriouſly to conſider, and by induſtrious Courſe, of Life in the Ways of Virtiue by which he may advance and bring to light the Treaſures of his Soul, and good Talants the Lord hath indued him with; Idleneſs being a greater Evil then moſt imagines; it breaks the firſt Command of God, and contradicts the whole Courſe of Nature, and is the Mother of Oppreſſion and Violence; a Sin that never goes alone, but attended with a black Train of Vices, always ſubject to the groſs inferiour Powers and evil Demons, which continually prompt him on to commit all kinds of Outrages againſt God and his Law in Nature, and iſ thc firſt to all Evils.

There is a reſerved Opinion amongſt, not only both ignorant Country-men, but even thoſe that pretend to Learning, that at the latter end of Summer, about *Michaelmaſe*, that the Sap or Eſſential Vietue in Trees, does fall down or retreat into the Root, and at the return of the Sun in the Spring it aſcends again, and repleniſhes the Tree, and all its Branches. But this is a very fond, tho almoſt gcneral Error; for if this were true, the Roots of all Trees would be indued with a far greater quanity of Juice or Radical Moiſture in the Winter than in the Summer, whereas the contrary is moſt evident, *viz.* That there is nothing near ſo much Juice Moiſture, or Sap in the Roots of Trees in the Winter as there is in Summer, or at lealt wiſe not ſo much manifeſted. The like iſ to be underſtood in the Body and Branches: I refer to any Artiſt, and let him ſeparate the Parts.

Beſides, there is a great Argument to confute this Error, (*viz.*) If the Sap that is the Radical Moiſture or Eſſential oyley Property, whence Life and Growth, Light and good Comeplexion of all Trees ariſe, and takes king, ſhould thus deſcend into the Root, and there inhabit all the cold Winter, then it were impoſſible that any of the reſt of the Tree ſhould live for when that Eſſential Vitue or Sap is withdrawn from any Tree, or part of a Tree, the ſame will immediately wither, rot, and periſh; Animal can as well live and ſubſiſt without Blood, as a Tree without Sap, or any part thereof, or of this oyley Moiſture: But moſt true it is, that at The Declining or Retret of the Sun, and Approach of Winter, this Eſſential Oyl or Sap doth every where Retreat into the main Body, or the, Root, but abſconds it ſelf inwardly in every Branch or Twig, and when it is ſtrong and vigorous, the cold and fierceneſs of the Elements cannot hurt it or the Tree, but of it be week or indiſpoſed, for want of ſufficent or due Noriſhment from the Earth in the Summer before, then the Severity of the Seaſon prevails upon it, and extinguiſheſ it, and forthwith ſuch Twigs, Branch, or Tree dies and no aſcending Sap they talk of from the Root can revive it; but if it withſtands the Winter rigor by virture or Radical Mits Internal Virtue or Radical oiſture, then as ſoon as the glorious Eye of the World, and natural Parent of Life, returns towards our Zenith, with his cheriſhing Beams and ſweet Influences, the ſame is ſet at Liberty, and opens Natures Priſoners; unlocks the Doors, and opens the Paſſages, and chaſes away the cold Saturnine Air, and warms every thing, and makes it Buxom, Jocond and Active, and by ſimile kindles and awakens all the chill, ſleeping, good qualities, and incorporating its own Virtues, invites abroad the Sap or oyley Moiſture from the Center, and mildly draws it forth to the ouermoſt Parts and Extremities of every Bough, and ſo tis puſht on to a further Growth, and ſpruces it ſelf up in Leaves, and

Bloſſoms, and Fruits according to its Kind.

AN

EXPERIMENT

For keeping of

EGGS.

THo it may ſeem forreing to the Matter, yet I ſhall (take this Opportunity) advancing to Communicate to the World another Notion, which I perſwade myſelf not commonly known.

That Eggss are an exellent ſort of Food, both by themſelves raw, eaten with good

Bread, being the beſt way, and to the greaſt advantage; and aſlo they ſerve to make up ſeveral ſorts of Spoonmeats and Diſhes, no Body can deny; and great improvement might be made of them by Perſons that go long Voyages to Sea, were it not that they have been told they will not keep. The truth is, we find moſt of the Eggs that are brought from *Scotland* or *Ireland* are muſty by that time they arrive here.

But I muſt crave leave to ſay, that it isnot the time, but the ill keeping of them that makes them naught, I mean, becauſe they are crowded up in Holes and cloſe Veſſels and debarred from the Air; for I have kept Eggs three, four, or five Months lying open upon a Shelf, or the like, in an open airy Room, and proved as good as it but new laid; and, as I doubt not but any Body may do the like, ſo I am apt to think, they may hold good at Sea, tho in hot Climates, if you afford them Air enough, full as long, nay perhaps for ſix or ſeven Months, which might eaſly be done by contriving Wicker Baſkets with ſeveral Stories or Frames one above the other, and between, on which the. Eggs might lye one by one without danger of breaking, and ſo might many times be expoſed to the briſk Air on the Decks, and at other times ſet in Cabbins. Thus any Man that loves not Salt Sea Diet (moſt apt tp breed the Scurvy) may victual himſelf with two or three hundred of Eggs for a Voyage. Thus Eggs might be brought out of *Scotland* (not to be ſold as now they are cried, Twelve a Groat, when they are good for nothing, and you cannot have above half ſo many good ones for that Mony) but,at a good Rate, and prove a profitable Commodity Theſe alſo, poor Houſe-keepers, might about Hatrveſt ſend in to the Country, when Eggs are Twelve a groat, and lay ın three or four hundred of them for all the Winter as good Huſbands do Butter and Cheeſe. I am ſure, if you let them have Air , they will keep good four, five or ſix Months, and probably longer. I ſhall inſiſt no further on this Matter, the ingenious open Trial will be able to judge whether it may not prove of confiderable advantage to divers Perfons.

The Natural Way how every one may in the Spring and Fall purge themfelves with Eafe add Pleafure to confiderable Advantage, with the Common Sallad and Herbs that are generally eaten in thefe Seafons, and alfo with Roots. One Example will ferve for all.

TAke much *Spinage* as Will go into a two Gallon Veffel, unto which add one Pint of Water, then ftew it with the faid Veffel uncovered when it is almoft prepared, add only Salt to it, then difh it up, and drik the Broth, and eat the Herbs freely with Bread, with out either Butter or other Fats; make your Dinner of thes Herbs two or three days together, as you ſhall find them more or leſs Operate or Purge. The very ſame Method you may uſe with other Herbs, either Simple or Compound, and alſo with Roots *viz.* Take Turneps, cut them ſmall, then ſtew or boyl them as you do the Herbs, drink the Broth, and eat the Roots with Bread and Salt, without any other Addition, and they will have the ſame Operation; but you muſt obſerve to eat Watergruel Morning and Night, into which you muſt not add any Ingredient, only Bread and Salt, and made according as we have taught in our *Monthly Obſervations for Health*; and thoſe that do not like ſtewed Herbs or Roots, may boyl them, obſerving the ſame method of eating them, and drinking the Broth, and ſo they will in all Reſpects anſwer your Deſires, and Purge you both by Urine and Stool, to your great Satiſfaction, far better than moſt of the Potions and Purges preſcribed by the Learned, which for the moſt part are not only Forreign, but Compounded of things of a agreeing Nature; but our own Herbs and Roots, thuſ prepared and eaten, are excellent as well in preſerving of Health, aſ preventing Diſeaſeſ, *viz.* by aſſiſting Nature to throw them off, when they have invaded the Body; in particular, they are profitable againſt the Stone or Gravel, and griping Pains of the Bowels, by diſburthening Nature of ſuch ſuperfluous Matter, and keen ſharp Juices that cramp the Body, they alſo cleanſeth the Stomach and Veſſels the thereof, which are generally ſtopt and furr'd by the frequent eating of Fat, ſucculant Food, and ſtrong Drinks, but the uſe of theſe Herbſ does cool and remove the Obſtructions that lie in the Paſſages, preventing Fumes and Vapors from flying into the Head, cleanſeth the Blood, cauſing it to circulate freely, and chearſ the Spirits, making the Body briſk and lively, being alſo profitable againſt ſhortneſs of Breath, Phlegm, and all Watery or Dropſical Hourmours, more eſpecially if Order and Temperance be obſerved; for the beſt Means or Medicines cannot but prove ineffectual when Diſorders, and the ſame Intemperances are continued, which were the firſt Originals of the Diſeaſe, moſt Diſtempers being contracted thorough Exceſs and Innordinate Living, nor doth any thing preſerving the Body, and alſo the Mind in Health ſo much as Sobriety and Temperance in Meats, Drinks, and Exerciſes, and not to heap together Superfluity of various ſorts of rich Compounded Foods and ſtrong Drinks of diſagreeing Natures beyond the Neceſſity, or truly the Digeſtive Power of Nature. The ancient Wiſemen that lived to great Ages in perfect Health, were contented with ſimple Food and mean Drink, and would be our Happineſs to Imitate them. I wiſh I might be an Inſtrument to perſwade my County-men to ſuch Moderation; and in order there unto I do recommend the uſe of the fore mentioned Herbs and Roots, and alſo to theſe following Obſervations.

A Method how every one may with Eaſe and Pleaſure keep their Body open, and prevent Coſtiveneſs, and being too much bound in their Bodies.

TAke *Spinage*, *Sorrel*, or ant other Herbs uſaually eaten in raw Sallads, eat them freely every day at Dinner, or every other day raw with your Bread and Butter, and Cheeſe or Bread and Fleſh, and they will certainly keep your Body open, and in brave, briſk, lightſom Condition, but remember that you eat them as they come from the Garden, without either Salt, Vinegar, or Oyl, for this Compoſit ion fixes them, that their genuine Nature, or friendly opening, mild qualities are not felt; few are ſenſible of the power of Compoſitions, and how it alters and changes moſt things for the worſe, more eſpecially when the Ingredients are of contrary Natures. And thoſe that deſire to underſtand more this, may read our *Way to Health, long Life, and Happines,* where they may have Satisfaction. Alſo Herbs thus eaten, do not only keep the Body in a due Temperature, but they mightily help Concoction, making all ſorts of hard Food, eaſie in the Stomach, preventing Fumes and Vapors, eſpecially if a Glaſs of our thin cold Gruel be drunk, ſo ſoon aſ you have dined, which you may find taught in our *Monthly Obſervations for Health.*

FINIS.

Made in United States
Troutdale, OR
11/03/2026

56844700R00073